THE BRONX DIET

by Richard Smith

**Workman Publishing
New York**

Jacket and book design: Paul Hanson
Jacket photo: Jerry Darvin
Illustrations: Marty Norman

Workman Publishing Company
1 West 39th Street
New York, New York 10018

Manufactured in the United States of America
First printing February 1979

10 9 8 7 6 5 4 3 2 1

Library of Congress Cataloging in Publication Data

Smith, Richard
    The Bronx Diet
    Bibliography: p.

    1. Reducing diets—anecdotes, facetiae, satire, etc.
    2. Diet—anecdotes, facetiae, satire, etc.
I. title
RM222.2.S623   613.2′5′0207   78-7320
ISBN   0-89480-063-9

Excerpt on pages 95-96 from *The James Beard Cookbook*. Copyright © 1959 by James A. Beard. Reprinted by permission of Dell Publishing Co., Inc.

FROM RICHARD SMITH, AUTHOR:

For over twenty years, I'd been trying to cope with my weight. There was no diet I hadn't been on, no pill I hadn't taken. I was a favored guest at reducing spas throughout the United States and Switzerland. To avoid the taste of pasta, I had my jaw wired shut. To avoid the smell of cooking, I had my nose wired shut. But the pattern remained the same. I'd start a new diet, enjoy extraordinary weight fluctuation on the first day, then go back to normal. It was no use. I couldn't control my eating habits and the prospect of forsaking my favorite foods drove me to despair. To begin the day without sponge cake, spend lunch hunched over a carrot, and eat a dinner lacking peanuts was worse than a prison sentence.

Then, one morning, I came across an article discussing a new diet being researched by a group of volunteer eaters in the Bronx. They referred to it as the "Eat all you want yet never be hungry" diet.

I took the subway 126 blocks to my first appointment. Eight days later, after following the regimen prescribed (except for tamale puffs), I discovered that my pants fit remarkably, yet I didn't feel as though I'd spent the last quarter of a month on a diet. My attitudes about food hadn't changed, I had eaten pretty much what I wanted and, best of all, experienced no feelings of deprivation or guilt, despite the inferior dumplings.

I'd like to share this revolutionary diet breakthrough with you.

Books by Richard Smith
_____

The Dieter's Guide to Weight Loss During Sex
The Bronx Diet

To my first eating tutor, who revealed to me the secrets of no-fault dieting.

"O, that this too too solid flesh would melt ... "

ACT I, SCENE 2
HAMLET

"Bring on the eats!"

ACT I, SCENE 1
BAR MITZVAH OF SID BORENSTEIN

CONTENTS

Introduction 11

What is the Bronx Diet? 14

I. UNDERSTANDING FOOD: IS IT REALLY FATTENING? 17

Evolution of Eating Food and Dieting 19
How We Use Food 21
Food and the Arts 23
Which Foods Are Genuinely Dietetic? 25
Why Some Foods Taste Better Than Others 26
Enhancing the Taste of Food 27
How the Appetite Works 28
Tongue Reflexology 29
How the Body Uses Food 30
How Food Affects Health 31
Why the Vitamins and Minerals Found
in Food Are Good for Us 32

II. EATING: IS IT REALLY GOOD FOR YOU? 35

Why We Eat 36
How We Eat 37
What Is Overeating? 38
What Is Undereating? 39
What Is Compulsive Eating? 40
The Nutritive Maze 41
The Art of the Dietetic Binge 42
What Is Compulsive Non-Eating? 46
What Do Compulsive Non-Eaters Eat? 47
Why Some People Are Underweight 48
Why Some People Are Overweight 49
Additional Reasons for Underweight 50
Additional Reasons for Overweight 51
What Are the Symptoms of Underweight? 52
What Are the Symptoms of Overweight? 53
Dangers of Underweight 54
Danger of Overweight 55
Advantage of Underweight 56

Your Ideal Weight 57
How Many Calories in the Ideal Human Being? 60
Is Your Figure Right for You? 61
How Body Weight Affects the Energy Crisis 62

III. WHY MOST DIETS FAIL 65

Why Bronx Is Best 66
Profile of a Well-Adjusted Eater 68
Profile of a Maladjusted Dieter 69
Drawbacks of Dieting.................................... 70
Typical Stages in the Life of a Non-Bronx
   Dieter While on a Non-Bronx Diet 71

IV. THE BRONX DIET: A DIET YOU CAN LIVE WITH 73

Rules of Eating—The Bronx Dieter's Creed 75
No More Guilt 76
Maintenance 77
Cheating 78
When Do You Go Off the Bronx Diet? 79
New Hope for Poor Eaters 80
Notice How Happily Your Body Responds 81
The Bite Report: Bronx Dieting and the
   Perfect Relationship................................. 82
Sex and the Bronx Diet 84
Training for the Bronx Diet 85
Defying the Bronx Diet 87
How to Follow the Bronx Diet 88
Before Beginning the Bronx Diet 94
What You Will Need to Go on the Bronx Diet 95
Proper Attire for the Bronx Diet 97
Foods Prohibited When on the Bronx Diet 98
Skipping, a Radical Concept 99
Substituting...100
How Much Food Should You Consume? 101
What to Do as You Approach Your Ideal Weight 102

V. THE BRONX DIET MEAL PLANS 103

Self-Punishment 106

Reward 108
Depression 110
Sex 112
Guilt. 114
Watching Television 116
Insomnia 118
Fatigue 120
Loneliness 122
Hangover 124
Courage 126
Boredom 128
Despair 130
Affection 132
Anger 134
Healthy Body Heat. 136
The Bronx Dieter's Guide to Dining Out 138

EPILOGUE: Final Thoughts for the Bronx Dieter 141

BIBLIOGRAPHY 143

THE RISE OF CIVILIZATION

- The Wheel
- The Steam Engine
- Electricity
- Indoor Plumbing
- Einstein's Theory of Relativity
- Freud's Theory of Relatives
- Penicillin
- Air Conditioning
- UFO's
- The Bronx Diet

INTRODUCTION

"Outside of every thin person, there's a regular-size person scream-ing to get in."

                                                    ANON.

Today, eating is America's fastest growing sport. The National Eater's Association estimates that there are over 200,000,000 eaters in the United States and their ranks are growing con-stantly. As a result of this eating boom, dieting—the act of weight control through sorrow—has become America's second-fastest growing sport and, speculates one expert, there may soon be more dieters than eaters.

But just what is the ideal diet? Since the Renaissance and Leonardo da Vinci's invention of the bathroom scale, the perfec-tion of a sane system of eating—one that addresses the question: "How can I enjoy ziti casseroles and still wear snazzy jeans?"—has been a major goal of science. Beginning with Henry VIII's Workingman's Diet in 1534,* over 28,000 diets have been de-vised, all promising mastery over our weight.

Unfortunately, the success rate for most of these diets is, to say the least, dismal. Last year, for example, of the 68,543,023 Americans who began some kind of diet, 68,543,015 experienced hunger pangs within the first 12 minutes and only 8 actually held their weight down long enough to trade in their pants.

To be sure, in the beginning stages of most industrial-strength diets, the dieter does lose pounds, frequently in spec-tacular quantities, and truly assiduous dieters, during the first weeks of a crash diet, have been known to drop a hat size. Inevitably, however, the body rebels, and the demand for normal nourishment such as peanut butter and muffins becomes over-whelming. Predictably, the efforts of even the most resolute dieter collapse, the first stages of cheating begin, and he helplessly orders Perrier with a twist of cupcake.

The problem, of course, is not the dieter but the diets, most of which tell us to ignore our natural eating abilities and "reach for a carrot instead of a fruit mousse," an act that is certain to cause

---

*On which Ferdinand Magellan shed 62 pounds while circumnavigat-ing the globe.

asthma. The people devising these diets are generous with their theories concerning what they term "food abuse." One doctor, who bases his diet on radio waves, insists that eating more than 800 calories a day is necessary only for those who are hunters and gatherers. Another, whose Veal Through a Straw diet achieved brief popularity, asserts that eating is merely a hedge against starvation. And finally, in what may be the most radical theory of all, a maverick clinician states that people unduly fond of eating were probably deprived during infancy, when they were nursed by an unskilled nanny through a sweater.

New studies, however, reveal that one's eating habits, like hair coloring or height, may be genetically determined and therefore unalterable. A love of corned beef hash with French fries, for instance, is inherited from a grandfather possessing a corned beef gene. An aversion to vegetables could be a family trait, traceable to an ancestor who was force-fed turnips by Cossacks. Indeed, most eaters unanimously insist that they never had to acquire a taste for spumoni or spaghetti carbonara but rather trusted their instincts, sat down and got right to work. Truly able eaters suggest that they were prodigies, easily coping with the rigors of goulash and shortbread well before the age of three.

It therefore becomes obvious that dieting is too important to be left in the hands of doctors, since any regimen asking us to tinker with our eating gifts is bound to cause a character disorder. A diet should consider the dieter, and that's what the Bronx Diet is all about.

ORIGINS OF THE BRONX DIET

The Bronx Diet came about in the spring of 1978, when a group of chronic dieters converged at the corner of Fordham Road and the Grand Concourse to protest the opening of another "fast diet" establishment, a radical weight loss clinic where dieters who cheated were thrown from a window. All of the protesters were victims of hundreds of diets that promised to "change their lives and firm their hips." For one dieter, high school student Clarence A., a varsity eater who had won his letter in the cafeteria, it was the third month on a Nine-Day Wonder Diet, which consisted mostly of juice and barley. True, Clarence had lost 70 pounds, but was finding it increasingly difficult to spell simple words and tie a bow. Another victim, Sophie J., had traveled down from Scarsdale where, after three weeks on a new "chemical reaction" diet, she complained that a strange reaction between grapefruit and carp had caused her to forget the names of her grandchildren. Ivan M., an ironmonger, after switching from beer and knishes to black coffee and salad, began hearing gongs. His girlfriend, Ellen X., changed her midnight snack from cookies to celery and found herself too weak to dream.

As the group exchanged diet stories, a question emerged: Why must weight control involve calories, carbohydrates, chemicals and scales—might it not be possible to control one's weight simply with food?

Experimental eating began immediately, based on a radical concept: to lose weight, eat less; to gain weight, eat more; if you merely wish to maintain, do whatever you were doing. The group then went even further, pulling dieting from the Dark Ages by constructing a scientific yet effective series of meal plans—a legitimate system of food therapy showing why food *should* be used as a crutch and which foods could be most effective in promoting spiritual and emotional satisfaction. For the first time, an eater could instantly grasp the connection between relieving depression and Mallomars, and understand why a lover's quarrel isn't so bad if there's a pint of ice cream nearby.

Results, to say the least, were phenomenal. Within three weeks, 31 members of the group had lost weight; nine members, all of whom had been unsuccessfully seeking voluptuousness, gained weight (including one 26-year-old anorectic who had plunged to 19 pounds); and 20 members of the group maintained their weight, fluctuating less than 1.5 grams. More significant, perhaps, was that nobody felt deprived, unloved or hungry and, best of all, the cholesterol count of every single person remained the same!

WHAT IS THE BRONX DIET?

A. The Bronx Diet is based on the theory (proven) that quantities of food are more important than the chemical reaction between them. To be sure, a steak reacts more favorably with red wine than with a malted, but this is an exception.

Q. Could you elaborate?
A. Yes. The Bronx Diet holds that we all need nourishment to go to work, wash the car, do a laundry, and sit up straight. That nourishment should relate with our particular personality, mood, and the activity involved. Nobody can build a brick wall with just a head of lettuce for lunch. Most diets, however, demand that we eat gloomy foods. The result is depression, loss of energy and paranormal experiences.

Q. How can I avoid depression, lost energy, and paranormal experiences?
A. By shunning any diet that asks you to change your eating habits and give up creature comforts such as cheesecake and ice cream.

Q. Aren't cheesecake and ice cream fattening?
A. Not if you're careful.

Q. And the Bronx Diet lets me eat whatever I want?
A. Pretty much.

Q. Whenever I want?
A. That, too.

Q. What about using food as a crutch? All diet books say it's wrong.
A. No, it's right. Food is a legitimate and happy substitute for misery, anxiety, bad sex, and a boring Monopoly game. Why should you suffer when there are Tootsie Rolls within reach? If you had a toothache, you'd reach for a painkiller, wouldn't you?

Q. And the Bronx Diet helps me control my weight?
A. Absolutely. It's all up to you. The Bronx Diet is what *you* want to make it. It has an "open end" feature permitting you to lose, gain, or maintain according to how much you take in. Eat what

you want when you want, following the Bronx Diet principles. You control your weight instead of a doctor under contract to a publisher.

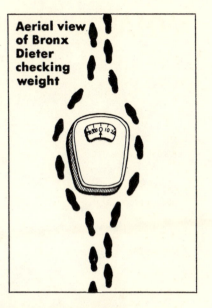

Aerial view of Bronx Dieter checking weight

Q. How often should I weigh myself?
A. Almost never. It makes things too confusing. See diagram at right for proper weighing technique.

Q. Will the Bronx Diet help me perfect my eating technique?
A. Yes.

DON'T PROCRASTINATE! START TOMORROW.

Here, then, is the Bronx Diet, a weight control plan that succeeds because:

•You don't alter your eating habits, and function therefore as a normal, happy person.

•It's easy to follow. Prescribed foods are always at your fingertips, whether you're in a French restaurant or a chili joint in Alaska.

•You're never embarrassed when dining out—dinner companions never suspect that you're on a rigid diet.

•There's never a feeling of deprivation. Feel sorry for yourself only when the bakery closes for inventory.

•It's inexpensive. If you can't afford expensive cuts of fish, try corned beef hash.

•You set your own goals—you have only yourself to blame for hunger pangs.

•You never go off the Bronx Diet, it's a way of life!

I.UNDERSTANDING FOOD: IS IT REALLY FATTENING?

Why is soybean curd less jolly than fudge? Are mung beans atrocious? Should a diver eat flanken? Despite the hundreds of food books published each year, our knowledge of food remains, at best, rudimentary. Certainly there is no dearth of facts. We are aware, for example, that excessive olive intake causes puffy eyes, that even ruffians weep over perfect linguine and that canned smelts are great for picnics. And even marginal eaters praise the healing powers of peanut butter. Yet, as 28,000 diets suggest, we are still in the dark as to the precise relationship between food, swallowing, and an impudent waistline. In this chapter, we will shed new light on food: what it is, what it can be, and why it should be an integral part of our daily diet.

"Great eaters are born with silver spatulas in their mouths."

EVOLUTION OF EATING FOOD AND DIETING

"The practice of eating food is as old as mankind, even older if we consider the amoeba."

PARAMECIUM

VERY EARLY PERIOD

Due to poor facilities, namely no running water or spoons, early man's diet* is pitifully basic, consisting of little more than roots and berries. For dessert he eats twigs. Later on, man discovers fire and perks up his menu with badger steaks, stews, and a primitive form of Rice-A-Roni. Pies and cakes are a rarity, served only on special occasions such as birthdays, weddings, and e-clipses. Little attention is paid to overweight, underweight, and tummies. Skinny medicine men and tubby warriors are accorded equal respect. A woman with cellulites is considered a good catch.

EARLY PERIOD

In May of 3000 B.C., the Sumerians invent the place mat and people find new ways to enjoy their food—for pleasure, business lunches, and surviving a rough divorce. As food grows more popular, people begin to nosh, especially during the holiday season. Tailors amass fortunes from letting out loincloths.

MIDDLE PERIOD

Dividing the day's nourishment into "meals"—breakfast, lunch, high tea, supper, and midnight snack—introduced by Charlemagne. Concept of ethnic food arises. Chinese food, for instance, begins to turn up in China and, to no one's surprise, French food in France. Weight control not yet understood and dieters are burned as heretics.

LATE MIDDLE PERIOD

Industrial Revolution in full swing, finally enabling the efficient

*Early woman's too.

production of little five-farthing pies and cakes, prototypes of today's Twinkies, Ring Dings and Devil Dogs. Groundwork is laid for the perfect, between-meal snack.

TODAY

A golden age of eating. More foods to choose from—mix 'n match pecan twirls, color-coordinated gravy, spaghetti available in individual strands—than ever before. The staggering variety provides unbounded opportunities for efficient and painless weight control without resorting to diets that distort reality.

LATER ON TODAY

The Bronx Diet.

"Thou shalt not covet thy neighbor's cooking aromas."

HOW WE USE FOOD

FUEL FOR THE BODY. As a source of energy, food is better than the sun and far more tasty. Food should be selected to complement a particular activity: two candy bars provide an avid stickball player with more pep than a bowl of leeks; a can of beer is nice when mowing the lawn; midnight snacks give us the strength to sleep until morning, and a glass of enriched gin (martini) is indispensable during an after-dinner speech. As an after-school pick-me-up, most children, exhausted from recess, thrive on milk and cookies.

PLEASURE. Most diets claim that pleasure should derive from sources other than food. This is obviously wrong, since a government survey of several thousand Americans put food second only to sex and golf as a major source of pleasure. (Third place was shared by having precocious children and finding a wallet.)

TO EXPRESS ANGER. Food can be used to express displeasure with a spouse, child, or live-in guest. Burned toast is subtle, but effective, as are mashed potatoes teeming with lumps and popovers filled with Di-Gel. An extreme case might be a platter of boiled chicken covered with lard. Imperfect sex partners can be punished with Cold Duck, hors d'oeuvres made with luncheon meat, and a reprimand.

PICNICS. Food is a great way to hold down the blanket.

RECIPES. Without food, most recipes would fail.

HEALING. Using food to make things "all better" began with the ancient Egyptians who cured headaches with a poultice of cheesecake. Today, principal among the healers are chicken soup, minestrone, and rum balls. Also in the "healing" category are beauty aids such as turkey legs for stronger nails, licorice for brighter eyes, and the carbonated face mask.

LOVE. Although certain misguided people try to "say it with flowers," the true language of love has always been food—a bouquet of roses is far less eloquent than a corsage of grapes. An edible symbol of affection can be nearly anything, from a simple square of rice pudding to a seven-course meal complete with candles, napkins, and a chair. A few further examples:

Love (passionate)	Golf-ball size truffles made from chocolate, butter and Grand Marnier; waffles with real maple syrup; homemade ice cream; peppercorn pâté; ripe brie; meat loaf with bacon on top.
Love (platonic)	Directions to a restaurant
Intense like	Croissants; Gruyére cheese; sacher torte; ratatouille; fettuccine Alfredo; beef Wellington.
Rapturous idolatry	Turkey leg; Beluga caviar; do-it-yourself lobster salad; coquille St. Jacques; chocolate-covered strawberries; Swedish meatballs.
Perfervid fascination	Garlic bagels; green sturgeon; home-fried potatoes; steak au poivre; roast goose with apple rings; Camembert.
Compulsive attachment	Soufflé-stuffed crêpes; kosher salami; filet of sole amandine; Chateau Margaux '64; turtles of giant almonds covered with imported chocolate; homemade lo mein.
Healthy devotion	Barbecued chicken; Russian black bread; imported beer; matzo brei; Milk Duds; cherry pie; corned beef and cabbage.
Hearty regard	Macaroons; French fried onion rings; hamburger; clam chowder.
Grudging admiration	Tuna fish on white; pigs' knuckles; *vin ordinaire*.

"If food be the music of love, eat on."

FOOD AND THE ARTS

LANGUAGE. Why is a bad actor called a "ham?" When angry, why do we threaten to make "mincemeat" out of someone? That we think about eating nearly as much as sex becomes evident in studying our language, which teems with allusions to food.

Ham radio

Chicken (coward)

Spring chicken (coed)

Grub stake

Apple of one's eye

Pie in the sky

Porkpie hat

Bowl of cherries (alternate definition of life)

Eat one's words

Eat crow

Pudding head

Bread (money)

Nuts ("He's nuts about her;" "Nuts to you!")

Lemon (a disadvantaged automobile)

Raspberry (Bronx cheer)

Cherry bomb (outlawed in some states)

Meathead

Duck! (get out of the way!)

Juice (electrical current)

Juicy ("That's a juicy story.")

Dough (money)

Doughy (complexion)

Butter up

Potato race

Cream (cream of the crop)

Baloney

Cheesy (a cardboard chair, for example)

Corny

One's salad days

Turkey ("That play was a real turkey.")

Pear shape

Lettuce (money)

Humble pie

Fruitcake (a person with amusing personality disorders)

Crab (ill-tempered landlord)

Tomato (the girl of one's dreams)

Date ("How about a date?")

Fish for a compliment

MUSIC. And, of course, America's obsession with food is clearly manifested in our musical heritage.

"I'm a Yankee Doodle Dandy"

"Tangerine"

"Sugar Blues"

"Don't Sit Under the Apple Tree with Anyone Else But Me"

"The Night They Invented Champagne"

"Beer Barrel Polka"

"I've Got a Lovely Bunch of Coconuts"

"Jelly Roll Blues"

"You're the Cream in My Coffee"

"Tea for Two"

"Comin' Through the Rye"

"The Jelly Bean Stomp"

"Strawberry Fields Forever"

"Honeysuckle Rose"

"Turkey in the Straw"

"Country Pie"

"If I Knew You Were Coming, I'd Have Baked a Cake"

"Sugar in the Morning"

"Meat Me in St. Louis"

PAINTING. Oranges, apples, cheese, and, of course, *Woman Ascending a Mousse* (M. Duchamp).

SCULPTURE. Chocolate Easter bunnies.

WHICH FOODS ARE GENUINELY DIETETIC?

In studying the diet literature, we note that even the so-called experts can't agree on which foods are dietetically beneficial. One diet champions bacon and sausage; another forbids both, instead advocating summer squash and kale, foods that cause an eating block. A well-known diet doctor suggests that meat hardens the arteries; another claims that deviled ham softens them. The befuddled dieter, at a loss, tries several diets at once, producing the infamous "yo-yo" syndrome and the mystical need for bratwurst.

Fortunately for Bronx Dieters, the situation is different. Because it is soundly eclectic, the Bronx Diet preaches that, with the exception of the carrot (best used as a cudgel), all foods are either fattening or non-fattening, depending on the eater's ingenuity.

In addition, scientific evidence shows that except for army rations, all foods are basically the same*—the atomic structure of a potato pancake and that of a hot dog are remarkably similar, only the hot dog has one free electron, which is why it reacts favorably with mustard.

> *"Avoid veiny crumpets."*

---

*Certainly there are minor differences. Pound cake is coffee soluble, Genoa salami is not. They also, at first glance, bear little resemblance to each other.

WHY SOME FOODS TASTE BETTER THAN OTHERS

Why isn't a bowl of spinach as satisfying as a bowl of chocolate mousse? What makes New England clam chowder more appealing than gruel? Why do we lick our fingers after spare ribs but never after aspirin? For centuries, the mystery of why some foods taste better than others has baffled not only science* but quite a few eaters as well. As we mentioned previously, the atomic structure of food, give or take a few electrons, is basically the same and, theoretically, there should be no significant difference between, say, apple strudel and Cheerios. Yet, evidence indicates that the typical eater will almost always opt for the apple strudel and sneer at the Cheerios.

"There's a big difference between 'health' food and 'healthy' food."

---

*A now-classic experiment in which an eclair and a rhubarb were placed side by side in a wind tunnel revealed nothing.

ENHANCING THE TASTE OF FOOD

Even more mysterious is why certain foods, when combined, taste even better. An alliance between rice and beans, for example, can produce a taste sensation that—weather permitting—will be felt just below the pelvis. Further examples of judicious food combining include:

Blintzes		Sour cream
Pie		Ice cream
Milk		Cookies
Liver	**GOOD**	Onions
Soup	⟵⟶	Crackers
Ham		Swiss cheese
Banana		Split
Slim Jims		Rolaids
Caviar		Champagne
TV dinner		Vitamins

Lox		Popsicle
Fudge	**POOR**	Whiskey
Jerusalem artichokes	⟵⟶	Seltzer
Oysters		Wheatena
Beets		Lorna Doones

	SILLY	
Pepperoni	⟵⟶	Smelts

HOW THE APPETITE WORKS

The human body contains trillions of cells, some craving oxygen, some craving pumpernickel. This cumulative craving is known as "appetite."* If your appetite works too well, you "overeat" and begin leaking soup.

> *"Why is it that the day before I start a diet, my cookie consumption triples?"*

*People with no appetite, therefore, have no cells.

TONGUE REFLEXOLOGY

An awareness of the relationship between food and the tongue is vital, for not only is the average tongue retractable, but within it resides a microcosm of our total being, including sections of the appetite. By manipulating pressure-sensitive areas of the tongue with food, we create "vibes" that affect the mind, body, and nearly every facet of our life. How this works is illustrated below.

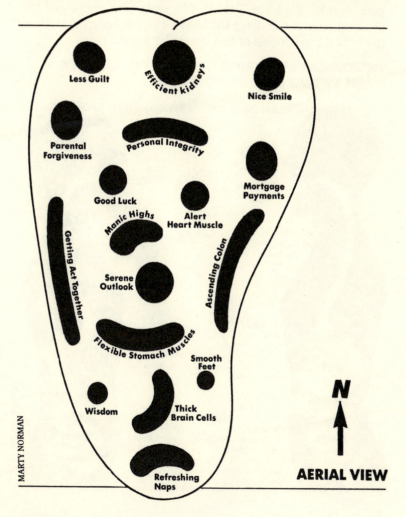

MARTY NORMAN

AERIAL VIEW

HOW THE BODY USES FOOD

What happens to the food we eat? The average eater, over the course of a lifetime, takes 3,576,006 bites of food, makes 24,885,042 chewing motions, swallows 6,863,567 times and uses 81,345 napkins. Yet, this average eater remains ignorant concerning the fate of food once it leaves the teeth. Certainly we know that milk builds strong bones, fruit expedites digestion and garlic wards off guests. But what happens after these and hundreds of other foods enter the body? The following chart details the typical trajectories of two dissimilar foods.

ANATOMICAL RENDERING OF DIGESTIVE JOURNEY TAKEN BY TWO CONTRASTING FOODS

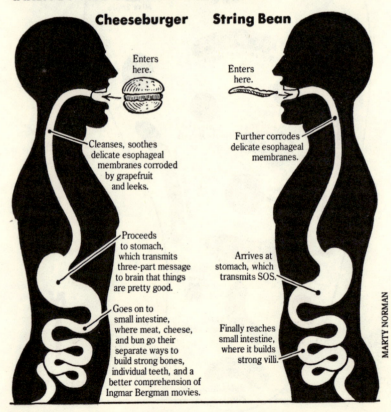

Cheeseburger

Enters here.

Cleanses, soothes delicate esophageal membranes corroded by grapefruit and leeks.

Proceeds to stomach, which transmits three-part message to brain that things are pretty good.

Goes on to small intestine, where meat, cheese, and bun go their separate ways to build strong bones, individual teeth, and a better comprehension of Ingmar Bergman movies.

String Bean

Enters here.

Further corrodes delicate esophageal membranes.

Arrives at stomach, which transmits SOS.

Finally reaches small intestine, where it builds strong villi.

MARTY NORMAN

HOW FOOD AFFECTS HEALTH

The concept of food therapy goes back to the 12th century when, to halt infection, wounded knights were given doughnuts. Today, millions consider food the universal healer, using it for everything from an emotional crisis (marzipan after five nights of horrendous sex) to easing the discomfort of stomach ulcers (sausage and peppers on date-nut bread).

The following chart presents but a few of the ways in which food has a positive effect on our physical and mental well-being.

AT-A-GLANCE FOOD THERAPY CHART

Affliction	Remedy
Unflattering haircut	Lemon Sherbet
Anxiety over job interview	Double scoop ice cream cone with sprinkles
Furniture repossessed	Pastrami on rye with mustard
Coughing and coughing	Gargle with tepid borscht
Rejection (by lover, Army, American Express)	Large pizza with extra cheese
Traffic ticket	Moussaka
Spotting a UFO	Deep-dish apple pie
Abuse by surly plumber	Brioche
Blind date resembles a pomegranate	Banana split and large container of bourbon
Corporate upheaval in which you get upheaved	Gingered crown roast of lamb and five Excedrins
Unresolved Oedipus complex	Milk and cookies
Frogbite	Chili
Impotence	Lox

WHY THE VITAMINS AND MINERALS FOUND IN FOOD ARE GOOD FOR US

SUBSTANCE	SOURCE	APPLICATION
Vitamin A	Chicken livers, carp, and mustard greens	Clears up acne and gastritis; banishes morning mouth; strengthens resistance to bullies; discourages clog dancing
Vitamin B	Seeds, yeast, and pumpkins	Denser hair, spiffier nails, perkier hips; also improves ability to negotiate peace treaties
Vitamin C	Florida	Fights the common cold, sometimes unsuccessfully; mitigates debilitating effects of Saturday night celibacy
Vitamin D	Cod-liver oil, mushrooms, and sunshine	Prevents teeth from wiggling and skin from sliding off; improves wardrobe coordination
Vitamin E	Wheat germ, roots, and breast milk	Nattier eyebrows, better sex life, richer orgasms; keeps the tummy flat during earthquakes

SUBSTANCE	SOURCE	APPLICATION
Niacin*	Goat's milk and luncheon meat	Keener vision, meaner tennis serve; hastens digestion of Serbian delicacies
Riboflavin	Cornstarch, roast chicken, and bread pudding with raisins	Repels gypsies and aluminum siding salesmen; helps you cope with est graduates
Thiamin	Egg noodles and immature cowpeas	Dispels erotic tension during funerals and business meetings
Iron	Calf's liver and girders	Winning attitude, stiff upper lip; prevents buildup of cholesterol in tear ducts
Bismuth	The ground	Controls naughty thoughts during Lent and Purim
Magnesium	Banana flakes and mature pigeon peas	Nature's own laxative
Chromium	Auto bumpers	Prevents embarrassing borborygmus
Plutonium	Bombs	Survive unexpected visits from neighbors and the Welcome Wagon

*Has been found to cause hemorrhoids in mice.

II. EATING: IS IT REALLY GOOD FOR YOU?

"When it comes to food, more is more."

Like breathing and dodging traffic, eating is instinctive, a lifelong habit that starts in the womb, where precocious eaters demand gourmet baby food. As we get older, we witness the phenomenon of the mouth growing larger and an increase in our eating abilities. The average teenage mouth, unless stuffed with corrective rubber bands, should be able to accommodate 40 cubic centimeters of M&M's plus a 7-inch bagel with minimal distortion.* At the zenith of one's eating powers (usually between the ages of 20 and 86), there are ample opportunities to inhale Oreos, demolish drumsticks, and pop Jujubes without moving the lips.

Poor eaters, on the other hand, reveal their malady early, refusing to eat unless they're coaxed and bribed. The feeder, usually an irate parent, must then resort to the "One for Uncle Julius" system of inducement, a tedious and time-consuming process that tempts the parent to tip over the highchair.

In this chapter, we will discuss some new facts about eating while correcting a few of the myths that have lately damaged eating's good name.

---

*In emergencies, a well-rounded eater should be able to dilate the mouth enough to conceal a jelly apple.

WHY WE EAT

What motivates a majority of the human race to take in food, to endure the daily drudgery of opening wide, chewing and swallowing, and then probing the teeth for particles? For years, eating masters have argued that a better understanding of why we eat would enable us not only to control our weight, but to actually eat more. Unfortunately, faulty diet research has given rise to numerous myths concerning our reasons for eating, the most prevalent being hunger, nutrition, and banquets. Now, however, a survey of 50,046 Americans who eat has shed new light on our gustatory habits, revealing several new and previously unexplored eating incentives, among them:

- To keep digestion in tune.
- To show off.
- Patriotism (to help the farmer).
- Religious ritual.
- Toughens the throat muscles.
- As an escape from the pressures of starvation.
- To satisfy cravings for "a little something."
- As an erotic supplement to the sex act.
- To restore a failing appetite.
- Perk up tired lips.
- Ward off dizzy spells.
- Because children in Europe are starving.
- Companionship. (If you are lonely, a meal of fried chicken, corn on the cob, white wine, and pie is like having a best friend over.)
- To pass the time in Laundromats.
- To relieve shortness of breath.
- To relieve tallness of breath.
- Oral contraception.

HOW WE EAT

Tirelessly

Voraciously

Noisily

Wetly

Lovingly

Greedily

Heartily

Hungrily

Wholesomely

Foolishly

Abstemiously

Daintily

Gluttonously

Ravenously

Voluptuously

Prudently

Sloppily

Nutritiously

Willingly

Uncontrollably

"We are all members of the Salivation Army."

WHAT IS OVEREATING?

Since individual capacities vary, finding the precise meaning of "too much eating" may be like trying to define "too much sex." Both leave you limp and shaky but it doesn't seem to matter.

To one eater, overeating might be a stomach in traction after Thanksgiving dinner; to another, the need for oxygen after a mere three pounds of rice pudding. To make matters even more confusing, a noted food ethnologist, in a monograph entitled, "I Couldn't Possibly Eat Another Thing," contrasts a fabled race of pygmies with one-inch stomachs, unable to eat more than six Tic Tacs without feeling stuffed, with a Bulgarian horse-lifter who, after eating 150,000 units of luncheon meat, could still do justice to a vat of chopped chicken liver and a Pepsi.

The most common definition of overeating, accepted by certain physicians, is "any act of ingestion producing sweating and shivering" or, after eating a seventeen-course meal, pitching face forward into the cherries jubilee.

"On most diets, to feel full, the stomach must have a good imagination."

WHAT IS UNDEREATING?

Stuffing foods you don't like into the couch.

"Most diets are movable famines."

WHAT IS COMPULSIVE EATING?

Professional eaters define it as "not wasting a healthy appetite." Symptoms include placing more than two utensils in the oral cavity at once, eating candy bars without removing the wrapper, nibbling on waiters, and keeping a walk-in bread box next to the bed. The clinical definition of compulsive eating, according to a prominent figure authority, is an eater who follows the classic "Nutritive Triangle" to excess.*

NUTRITIVE TRIANGLE

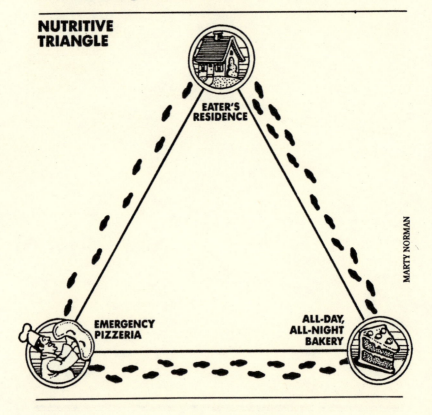

EATER'S RESIDENCE

EMERGENCY PIZZERIA

ALL-DAY, ALL-NIGHT BAKERY

MARTY NORMAN

*Seven or more times each day, in all kinds of weather.

THE NUTRITIVE MAZE

Here is an extreme example of what some term "compulsive eating," sometimes called a binge.

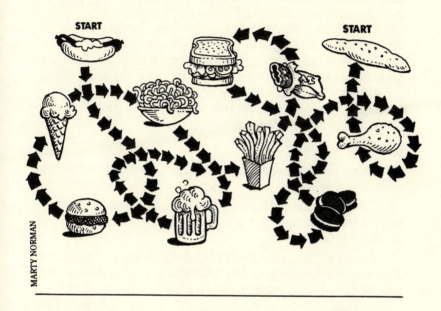

THE ART OF
THE DIETETIC BINGE

The map on the facing page traces the route of the first, explora-
tory Bronx Diet binge, a historic feat proving once and for all that
a binge could be thrilling and satisfying, yet dietetic.

It was during this seminal binge that our Bronx Dieter stum-
bled upon the technique of "painless moderation" when he discovered that one could easily avoid temptation by making no
superfluous detours. As we see on the map, the dieter simply
travels directly from one stop to the next, eating *absolutely
nothing* in between, thus preventing a modest eating adventure
from turning into a caloric spree.

LEGEND

1. Bronx Dieter, bewitched by food, but wishing to retain trim
good looks, sets out.

2. Stumbles upon the Sponge Cake Unlimited bakery where he
tests a charlotte russe for accuracy. Also orders a brownie but
doesn't eat the nuts.

3. Enters Forum of the Twelve Hot Dogs where he lingers over
a medium frank, paying no attention whatsoever to the one-cent
sale on French fries currently in progress.

4. At Lloyd's Chinese Restaurant dieter, after agonizing over
nine-page menu, decides on lo-cal but substantial order of shrimp
in lobster sauce; eats only half of his rice.

5. Reaches ice cream parlor and purchases lavish chocolate
cone. Exercising remarkable willpower, he denies himself fattening sprinkles.

6. Primed by the ice cream, dieter visits Lupo's Shake 'n Quake
House of Chili and Self Defense, samples small (12-oz.) bowl of
special fire chili. *Doesn't eat the crackers!*

7. Takes cab to Colonel Murray's Pizzeria where he has diet
pizza (no oregano), saving further on calories by leaving the
crusts.

8. Totters over to Italianissimo Angie's to check on the linguine

in white clam sauce. Avoids uncomfortable "stuffed" feeling by weeding out larger pieces of clam and donating them to a cat.

9. Concludes journey by droping in at Sam's All-Nite Deli ("beds on request") for a nightcap (size 7½) and to tamp down the day's eating with a pastrami and turkey on rye with cole slaw and Russian dressing. Demands thin-sliced bread.

10. Uncooked fish.

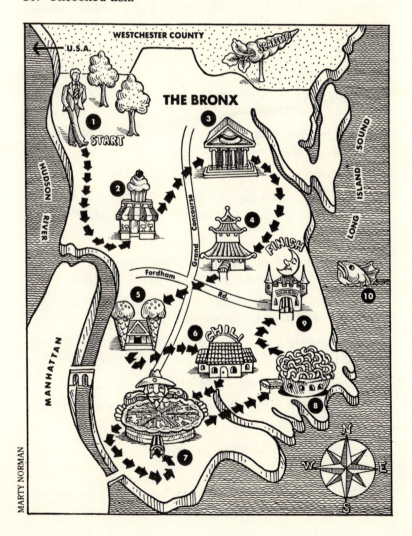

CREATE YOUR OWN BINGE

It isn't necessary to live in the Bronx to enjoy a Bronx Diet type of binge. The map on the previous page is meant only to guide you in planning an eating tour of your own area, no matter how remote from civilization it might be. For an example of a satisfying Bronx Diet dietetic binge that didn't occur in the Bronx, see below. The author, on location in a Nebraska hamlet, found it necessary to devise his own binge* upon discovering that the airline had lost the valise containing his food.

LEGEND

1. Hotel Room.

2. Candy machine down the hall. Purchases two Mounds bars but doesn't eat coconut.

3. Soda machine four feet to the right. Drinks little cup of Sprite. Strange beverage.

4. Hotel exit.

5. Dines al fresco on two souvlaki hero sandwiches. Contents fall into lap. Unusual but effective calorie-saving device.

6. Town square.

7. Bakery. Author eats three doughnuts. Removes the powdered sugar from each by holding against the wind.

8. Ice cream parlor. Buys pint of rum raisin but eats only half. Has to stop when plastic spoon snaps.

9. Haute cuisine fried chicken restaurant. Samples day's special: Bucket o' Giblets and all the noodles you can carry.

10. Texaco station. (Author gets lost.)

11. Mom and Pop and Brother and Sister grocery store. Orders three Devil Dogs to go.

*Technically a "bingette" due to a shortage of time and the author's unfamiliarity with the roads.

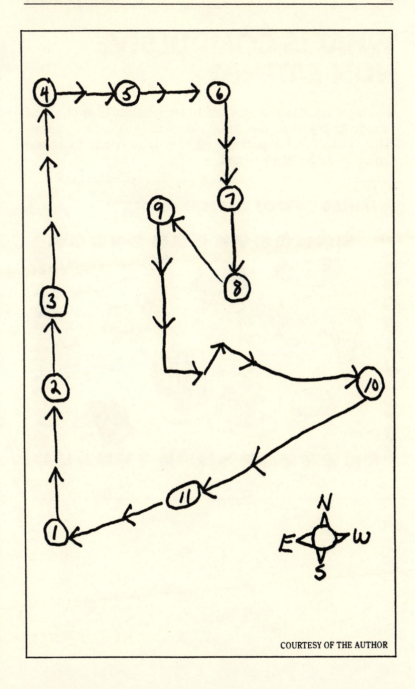

WHAT IS COMPULSIVE NON-EATING?

It usually begins as a hunger fast to protest conditions at a local zoo. Soon, however, the throat closes and the once voracious eater suddenly finds it possible only to swallow tidbits. In its final stages, an eating block occurs.

OVERHEAD VIEW OF AN EATING BLOCK

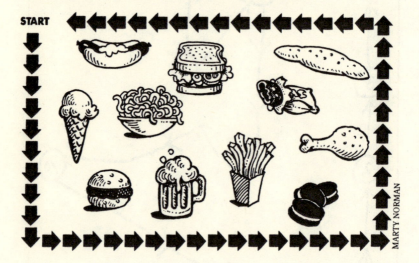

WHAT DO COMPULSIVE NON-EATERS EAT?

Despite hermetically sealed stomachs, even compulsive non-eaters find it necessary to take nourishment occasionally. But what do they eat? Cherry crumb pie? Chocolate swirl ice cream? Iced Fudgie cookies? Never. Preferred foods are those that either corrode or emit feeble pleasure waves. They include:

Tuna in water	Anchovy fillets
Herbs in solution	Asparagus
Wheat germ	Egg whites
Consommé	Abalone
Cottage cheese	Beets
Grapefruit	Bell peppers
Skim milk	Casaba melon
Decadent codfish balls	Boiled chicken
Celery	Protein toast
Broccoli	Spinach
Lettuce	Low-fat pot cheese
Pimentos (defatted)	Diet gelatin

"The road to ruin is paved with kelp."

WHY SOME PEOPLE ARE UNDERWEIGHT

As children, they rebelled against parental authority by eating leafy vegetables and flushing ice cream down the toilet.

"I tried the 'tiny bite' system of food control. It took two months to eat a banana."

WHY SOME PEOPLE ARE OVERWEIGHT

Similar situation except, as children, they flushed the leafy vegetables down the toilet and ate the ice cream.

"If one must take nourishment, it might as well be food."

ADDITIONAL REASONS FOR UNDERWEIGHT

- Too much nervous energy.
- Wacky bone structure.
- Reluctance to swallow food.
- Oral deficiency: mouth no larger than a dime.
- Citizen of India.
- Gullibility: believing a recipe when it says, "Serves two."
- Macrobiotic pork chops.
- Airline food.
- Brewer's yeast sandwiches.
- Ingesting the germs of wheat.
- Cookbooks written in Latin.
- Poor eating habits:
  - *Facing away from the table during mealtimes.*
  - *Chewing food too slowly (it stays in the mouth and evaporates).*
  - *Taking tiny bites (they get lost in the mouth and are never heard from again).*
- Eating soup while sitting on a moving tractor.

ADDITIONAL REASONS FOR OVERWEIGHT

• No metabolism.

• Large skin.

• Too many fattening salads.

• Fattening occupation: freelance guest at weddings and bar mitzvahs, for example.

• Sedentary regimen: going for long sits instead of long walks; moving the razor instead of your face; letting midgets shave your legs; using a messenger to water your plants or, worse, hosing down your plants from the couch.

• Drinking ale directly from the keg.

• Licking plates that don't belong to you, especially in restaurants.

"A Hostess Twinkie contains twice the restfulness as that found in a pound of calf's liver."

                                                    MARY HOSTESS

WHAT ARE THE SYMPTOMS OF UNDERWEIGHT?

You are carrying insufficient poundage if you:

- Slide through bench slats.
- Rise after jumping from a plane.
- Can't be seen.
- Have no contours.
- Are shy at orgies.

WHAT ARE THE SYMPTOMS OF OVERWEIGHT?

You are carrying excess poundage if you:

- Bend seesaws.
- Displace a volume of water equal to that of a Buick.
- Have difficulty jumping one inch into the air.
- Hide cookies in the folds of your skin.
- Have trouble breathing before climbing stairs.
- Dance without lifting your knees.
- Get winded from playing touch poker.
- Need a winch to enjoy sex.
- Rupture water beds.
- Can't sleep in a pup tent.
- Crush mopeds.
- Drink from heavy-duty goblets.

"My passion for fudge knows no bounds."
ARTHUR SCHOPENHAUER

DANGERS OF UNDERWEIGHT

- Lack of body heat.*
- Getting lost in elevators.
- A tendency to rise should gravity fail.
- Overexposure of bones to sunlight and gamma rays.
- Chickenesque appearance when naked.
- Wearing children's sizes when you're already in college.
- No resistance to wind.
- Inability to leave footprints.
- Skimpy shadow.

*This is why fashion models gravitate to hairy men with heaters in their car.

DANGER OF OVERWEIGHT

- Silly bowel movements.

ADVANTAGE OF UNDERWEIGHT

- Less work for the X-ray machine.

YOUR IDEAL WEIGHT

A major problem in determining ideal weight is the incredibly wide range of weights to choose from—anywhere from 95 to 360 pounds for the mature, fully formed adult. Complicating matters is the miraculous capacity of most human bodies to gain or lose weight, a trait which, even more than intelligence, separates so many of us from the vegetable kingdom.

Certainly there are any number of "Desirable Weights for the Average American" charts, but these have limited application due to a shortage of average Americans, especially in the Bronx and Utah. Most dieters will therefore find it easier, more accurate, and less frightening to calculate ideal weight by knowing what they *shouldn't* weigh.

"For best results, turn your bathroom scale over."

UNDESIRABLE WEIGHTS* FOR MEN, WOMEN, AND LARGE CHILDREN ‡

MEN

Height Feet	Inches	Small Frame	Medium Frame	Large Frame
6	6	90	92	94
6	5	93	95	97
6	4	94	96	98
6	3	95	97	99
6	2	96	99	101
6	1	99	101	102
6	0	100	102	104
5	11	103	105	107
5	10	105	107	110
5	9	260	274	290
5	8	255	270	275
5	7	240	262	268
5	6	230	236	241
5	5	225	230	235
5	4	75	79	81
5	3	68	71	73
5	2	50	52	56
5	1	45	47	68
4	6	164	180	200

WOMEN

| Height | | Small | Medium | Large |
Feet	Inches	Frame	Frame	Frame
6	8	84	86	88
6	6	86	87	89
6	5	83	85	87
6	4	81	82	80
6	3	90	92	97
6	2	95	96	98
6	1	99	99	99
6	0	102	103	107
5	11	80	82	84
5	10	71	68	66
5	9	68	71	73
5	8	65	67	70
5	7	51	53	55
5	6	172	174	177
5	5	176	180	184
5	4	180	180	180
5	2	41	45	47
5	0	39	40	41

*In pounds.
‡Adapted from actuarial tables prepared by Hank's Life Insurance Co., Inc.

HOW MANY CALORIES IN THE IDEAL HUMAN BEING?

A 160-pound man—with a wife and two children, perhaps the vice-president of a medium size corporation with a cheery financial picture—contains 530,000 calories, which is equivalent to the number of calories found in either 3,600 sugared crullers or enough celery, placed end to end, to reach from Scarsdale to the Bronx.

IS YOUR FIGURE RIGHT FOR YOU?

Before deciding how much to weigh, stand in front of a mirror and study your figure.* Are you short and wide, tall and narrow, mannish but womanly? Science tells us there are four body types, each with separate and distinct characteristics. Studying the classifications below will enable you to determine your particular body build, assess any structural deficiencies, and then select the weight most flattering to you.

1. Endomorph—Usually a round, soft, almost Rubenesque figure, curvaceous, slightly hippy (often not unpleasingly) and a fuller face (Dolly Parton, Mario Lanza, Sophie Tucker, Benito Mussolini, Sophia Loren, Babe Ruth, successful maharishis).

2. Mesomorph—Generally well-proportioned, squarer type of figure, athletic and muscular, with narrow hips, broad shoulders, noticeable bust (Arnold Schwarzenegger, Bunnies, Ann-Margret, drill instructors, Johnny Carson, Spring Byington, Henry Winkler, Southern cheerleaders).

3. Ectomorph—Smaller, fashion-model, more angular type of figure, with thinner arms and legs, small hips, narrow chest and often imperceptible bust (Mick Jagger, Sandy Duncan, Shirley Temple [preteen], David Niven, Tutankhamun).

4. Morph—Not too fat, not too thin, not too tall, not too short, yet curiously not just right. Morphs manifest a marked aversion to food and ribald behavior, possibly because their ancestors came over on the Mayflower (John, Priscilla, Miles, et al.).

---

*That part of the body directly below the face. If you haven't a mirror, just look straight down.

HOW BODY WEIGHT AFFECTS THE ENERGY CRISIS

A recent report indicates that Americans, altogether, are 2.3 billion pounds overweight and, by eliminating excess bulk, could save the nation the equivalent of more than a billion gallons of gasoline every year.

A billion gallons of gasoline is a trifling amount, however, since another report, using a more judicious accounting system, reveals that Americans, altogether, are also 3.6 billion pounds underweight and suggests that insufficient body bulk may actually be the bigger energy-draining villain:

• Thin people damage the economy, since the gasoline they save creates unemployment in the energy field (A town comprised of skinnies used so little gasoline that its four service stations went bankrupt.)

• Due to a lack of body bulk, thin people generate less body heat and therefore require more fuel to heat their homes.*

• Lack of body heat makes it necessary to wear warmer clothing such as wool and furs, thus causing the death of many innocent sheep and minks.

• Many of those deficient in body bulk require more light to read by, perhaps because their eyes are smaller.

• Because automobiles driven by thin people are lighter, there is less traction on snow and ice, making them accident prone.

• Preparing the foods eaten by thin people requires huge amounts of energy to prepare:

> • *The consumption of toast drains 197 million kilowatts of electricity every morning.*

---

*People with excess body bulk generate enormous amounts of energy-saving body heat, which actually saves energy. A 265-pound man, when excited, can easily heat a six-family dwelling.

• *The constant demand for yogurt and cottage cheese is sorely taxing the udder power of the nation's cows.*

• *It takes more square feet of dirt and fertilizer to grow a head of lettuce than it does to grow a candy bar.*

Thin people also have higher medical bills since their lack of thickness produces easily broken bones. (It is said that thin people have a thin sense of humor. This is because they're afraid to slap their thighs.)

HOW WEIGHT AFFECTS GAS MILEAGE

IF YOU ARE:	YOU SHOULD GET (M.P.G.)					
	FORD	BUICK	LINCOLN	TOYOTA	MASERATI	HARLEY DAVIDSON
90 to 100	21	15	12	24	3	94
110 to 120	20	14	11.4	23.6	2.9	93
121 to 130	19.5	13.5	11	23	2.6	92
131 to 140	18	13	10.7	22.4	2.4	90
141 to 150	17.7	12	10	22	2.2	87
151 to 165	17	11.7	9.5	21	2	85
166 to 180	16.3	11.2	9.1	20.8	1.9	83
181 to 195	16	10.7	8.7	20	1.6	80
196 to 210	15	10	8	19	1.3	78
211 to 225	14	9	7	18.4	1	76

TIPS TO INCREASE FUEL EFFICIENCY

• Avoid jackrabbit starts.

• Avoid frequent starting and stopping (go through stoplights).

• Siphon gas from your neighbor's tank.

• Pedal when convenient.

• Change your shoes every 10,000 miles.

III. WHY MOST DIETS FAIL

"Starvation takes the fun out of fasting."
                                        MAHATMA GANDHI

The average person eats 21 meals per week; the above-average person even more. Yet, by presuming that food causes weight problems, diet experts mistakenly devise eating regimens that shun brownies and corn bread, substitute melon balls for potato puffs and force the dieter to ingest items such as carrots, kelp,* and water-soluble meats. In extreme cases, the dieter, instead of losing weight, loses height and is forced to wear orthopedic pants sporting nine-inch cuffs.

As we can see from the Bronx Diet, however, food is not only innocent, but actually helps the dieter achieve weight control. After getting the hang of it, the Bronx Dieter walks around losing weight while enjoying such "forbiddens" as roast beef hash, little hot dogs in a blanket, and candy canes.

"The problem with most diets is their insistence on a Platonic relationship between the dieter and food."
                                        SOCRATES

---

*Causes squaring of the arteries.

WHY BRONX IS BEST

CONDITION OR AFFLICTION	RECOMMENDED ANTIDOTE	
	ATKINS	**SCARSDALE**
Anger	Bouillon	Protein toast
Boredom	Green pepper rings	Cooked spinach
Loneliness	One cup of salad (loosely packed)	Grapefruit (peeled)
Guilt	Diet soda	Salmon salad
Fatigue	Deviled ham and peppermint fizz	Coffee
Insomnia	Gelatin	Six walnuts
Sexual Dysfunction	Diet Revolution roll	Low-fat pot cheese
Despair	Stuffed celery	Cucumbers
Shingles	Lox	Cauliflower

RECOMMENDED ANTIDOTE

STILLMAN	MACRO-BIOTIC	DRINKING MAN'S	BRONX
Lean meat	Brown rice	Tom Collins	Cheeseburger with home fries
Leaner meat	Browner rice	Martini	Hazelnut torte
Clear broth	Brown rice	Gin toddy	Pizza
One peach	Tan rice	Whiskey sour	Ice cream
Any expensive cut of chicken	Fast	Brandy Alexander	Cheesecake
Lean fish	Herb tea	All of the above	Lasagna
Water (any kind)	Alfalfa	Harvey Wallbanger	Pastrami on rye with Fig Newtons
Young lamb chop	Fast	Bourbon	Brownies
Radishes	Chanting	Muscatel flip	Italian sausage with spaghetti

PROFILE OF A WELL-ADJUSTED EATER

- Practices defensive eating.
- Resides within staggering distance of a reputable take-out deli.
- Eats toast before it pops up.
- Eats with entire body and the mouth. Is proud of food stains.
- Registers hunger pangs with a seismograph.
- Refuses additional helpings only when there aren't any.
- Gets emotionally involved with food instead of seeing it only as a nutrition object.
- If necessary, can eat on an empty stomach.
- Laughs at utensils, especially at heavily populated smorgasbord tables.
- Eats between snacks.
- Doesn't lose his appetite during air raids.
- Enjoys airline food, even on the ground.
- Feels no guilt about leaving IOU's in empty ice cream containers.
- Uses food to turn ordinary experiences into great ones— television, reading, parking the car, and sex.
- Considers caviar inferior to a majestic Tootsie Roll.
- Eats salads and okra only by mistake.
- Keeps special foods in a refrigerated safe.
- Believes orgasm possible with the proper brioche.

"The true eater prefers that the cake be hidden inside the file."

PROFILE OF A MALADJUSTED DIETER

A dieter is nothing more than a lapsed eater who, by embracing various diets, commits various unnatural acts:

- Ignores hunger pangs.

- Maintains a brave front while enduring tortoni deprivation.

- Treats food as a nutrition object.

- Defaces ketone sticks.

- Feasts on water and meat. (Annihilates the taste buds and produces excessive chair-wetting.)

- Pretends that raw vegetables are peanuts and cake.

- Counts carbohydrates, calories, and molecules.

- Counts bites. (Difficult to do when drinking milk.)

- Eats by the ounce instead of by the mound.

- Resists the gravitational pull of ice cream and sticky buns.

- Puts in the mouth those things that are better left in the ground: celery, lettuce, roots, and mineral water.

- "Thinks thin." (Good only for those with a narrow head.)

- Puts food on a smaller plate "so it looks like more." (Works only for the simple-minded.)

"After three weeks on liquid protein, my husband didn't recognize me.
After six weeks, I didn't recognize my husband.
After nine weeks,

DRAWBACKS OF DIETING

The problems—emotional, physical, and social—with ordinary diets are highlighted in the following excerpts from interviews with disillusioned dieters seeking help at Bronx Diet Counseling Centers throughout the country.

"I've been on one hundred and twelve diets. First it was acupuncture. After putting needles through my appetite, I began obsessing over fortune cookies. Then I tried behavior modification. Instead of nibbling while watching television, the dietician told me to occupy my hands in a different way. So I took up woodcarving. The first week was fine, I made a walking stick. The second week, I binged and ate five pounds of oak."

DESPERATE

"On the Drinking Man's Diet I had trouble reading road signs. I also experienced difficulty when changing lanes, even while walking."

"I tried the carbohydrate diet and gained forty pounds. The drawback in counting carbohydrates is that they're so hard to see."

"Two weeks of Scarsdale reduced my cholesterol count to such a dangerously low level that I had to get emergency transfusions of fat."

"So much grapefruit triggered an abnormal reaction not only inside of my body, but several feet away from it."

"Why did my sexual performance plunge on Weight Watchers? Because, as my doctor explained, I was expending eighty-seven percent of my energy on willpower. The remaining thirteen percent was barely enough to survive foreplay."

"Going on someone else's diet is like wearing someone else's shoes."

TYPICAL STAGES IN THE LIFE OF A NON-BRONX DIETER WHILE ON A NON-BRONX DIET

FIRST DAY: Dieter awakens depressed. Feels abandoned by God and also very hungry. Temptation to procrastinate strong, especially with open carton of Mallomars on night table.

THIRD TO FOURTH DAY: Severe loss of energy due to cookie deprivation. Dieter collapses while attempting to scale side of refrigerator.

END OF FIRST WEEK: Lack of pasta and raisin bread create potash deficiency. Dieter experiences first wet food dream and awakens in a hot sweat. Periods of fatigue. Dieter frequently pitches face forward into bowls of consommé.

MIDDLE OF SECOND WEEK: Onset of sociopathic behavior. Instead of walking beloved dog, dieter merely holds it out the window.

END OF SECOND WEEK: Dieter discovered at 2:00 A.M. in compromising position with tea bag.

BEGINNING OF THIRD WEEK: Ravaging depression, possibly from grapefruit emissions. Telephones office and calls in dead. Dieter constantly licks his lips and those of other people, especially while they're eating. He's arrested twice and has his tongue impounded.

END OF THIRD WEEK: Dieter has shrunk to three feet, four inches and speaks in a chirp. Tries to prove he's Napoleon but poor command of French language* gives him away. In despair, dieter attempts suicide by sending himself a letter bomb.

MIDDLE OF FOURTH WEEK: Deep coma. Mirror held to dieter's mouth causes face to fog up.

*Dieter's knowledge of French limited to: *"un, deux, trois,"* and *"jai faim."*

IV. THE BRONX DIET: A DIET YOU CAN LIVE WITH

Like plague or dengue fever, most people regard dieting as an affliction. The Bronx Diet, however, because of its revolutionary principles, has been shown by test-eaters to be a regimen you can follow and enjoy for the rest of your life, even longer if you're careful.

In addition, the Bronx Diet, through its Meal Plans, gives you the advantage of a sane, sensible system of eating that runs the entire psychological gamut. For the first time in diet history, the eater can choose a meal to match and satisfy every mood and emotional state.

THE LAST DIET YOU'LL EVER NEED

The first thing you'll notice on the Bronx Diet is how easy it is to do the things you did before—visit favorite restaurants, swim, travel, or eat between meals—without the burden of that "I'm on a diet" feeling. Bronx Dieters, in fact, enjoy several eating-related activities that on ordinary diets would be unthinkable:

• A five-month veteran of the Bronx Diet, James T. (once a recluse, now a 41-long), with minimal training, took top honors in last year's Strudel Olympics at Lake Placid, New York.

• Helen R., snatched at the last minute from the jaws of vegetarianism, went on the Bronx Diet and spent her three-week vacation eat-tasting every recipe in Verona, Italy ... and she lost four pounds!

• Sir Albert Lortzing, an English Bronx Dieter, received his knighthood for being the first person to consume large quantities of British food without flinching.

• Leroy J. made 106 new friends at his "Eat All You Want Until You Fall on the Floor" free-eats party.

Additional activities permitted the Bronx Dieter include:

• In-depth sampling of almost every edible known to man, no matter what the altitude.

• Complete freedom of worship at any smorgasbord table.

• Unrestricted nutritive intake at all festive affairs—sales breakfasts, picnics, church socials, weddings, and bon voyage and Tupperware parties.

• Window shopping for bagels.

• Actually swallowing the wine at wine-tastings.

• Sneering at crisp green salads.

• Enjoying the free "happy hour" hors d'oeuvres until you go into shock.

• Toasting with a real drink. (Even the saintliest dieter would be hard pressed to enthusiastically toast a job promotion with bouillon.)

• Chewing.

RULES OF EATING — THE BRONX DIETER'S CREED

1. Never eat on an empty stomach.

2. Never leave the table hungry.

3. When traveling, never leave the country hungry.

4. Enjoy your food.

5. Enjoy your companion's food.

6. Eat at a comfortable pace—never more than one utensil in your mouth at a time.

7. Really taste your food. It may take several portions to accomplish this, especially if subtly seasoned.

8. Really feel your food. Texture is important. Compare, for example, the texture of a turnip to that of a brownie. Which feels better against your cheek?

9. Eat only in one room. Moving about creates air currents that will blow away your spaghetti.

10. Be sure to use a large enough table. It protects lap and shoes from falling objects.

11. Never eat between snacks, unless it's a meal.

12. Don't shop for food when you're hungry. You won't have the strength to carry it home.

13. Don't feel you must finish everything on your plate. You can always eat it later.

14. Avoid any wine with a childproof cap.

15. Avoid blue food.

NO MORE GUILT

"Your hands don't turn into flippers from touching candy bars."
ENLIGHTENED EATING INSTRUCTOR

Because the Bronx Diet supports our convictions about food—
that it is good for us and fun to eat—the Bronx Dieter is seldom
troubled by guilt, even after a four-napkin meal.

Ordinary diets, however, because they're based on repres-
sion, trigger guilt from the very first radish. Breaking any rule is
forbidden. For cookie-fits, hunger headaches, or a longing for
farfel, the dieter must drown his troubles either in broth or one
medium peach. Within a short time, the dieter, his natural im-
pulses inhibited by fear, manifests the classic symptoms of neu-
rotic guilt: hysterical fear of tacos, obsessive behavior in the
presence of lasagna, and late-night carrot circumcision.

It may interest the dieter to note that the following activities
and situations are considered to be the most guilt-inducing. On
the Bronx Diet, we are happy to report, they are considered
normal behavior for a vigorous eater:

- Gasping for breath after four helpings of pie a la mode.

- Eerie feelings in the teeth from eating many pralines.

- Rapacious ingestion of peanuts.

- Eating foods that defy the Geneva Convention: Czechoslova-
kian goulash; stew from diners named "Louie's"; ice cream with
122% butter fat content.

- Abnormal excretion of money when in bakeries.

- A post-Thanksgiving-dinner stuffed feeling, usually mitigated
by collapsing on a nearby couch or carpet, a drumstick still
hanging from the mouth.

- Split pants from sampling three of everything at Italian weddings.

- Wanton gulping of noodles.

MAINTENANCE

With most diets, "maintenance" is another term for lifelong death, a situation in which the dieter becomes a gastronomic shut-in, maintaining ideal weight by surviving on string beans disguised as French fries, sandwiches without the bread, and memories of healthier days. Even worse, the dieter—when upset or bored—has nothing to turn to but celery, flounder, and seltzer. This false eating produces a mysterious ailment known as "eating lag," caused by switching too abruptly from rigid dieting to semi-rigid dieting without that vital, "Let's celebrate my weight loss with ice cream" stage.

The Bronx Diet, with its built-in maintenance program, eliminates this problem since the dieter is actually maintaining from the very first day. Bronx Dieting becomes so natural that many dieters have been known to reach their ideal weight without even noticing.

"I've been on the Bronx Diet for twenty-six years. It's worked so well that I intend to leave it to my grandchildren."

Newton's Second Law of Eating: Anybody can gain weight. The trick is keeping it on.

CHEATING

On the Bronx Diet, since there are no prohibited foods (see page 98 for exceptions), there is no cheating.

On ordinary diets, because so many essential foods are taboo, the dieter, upon reaching the breaking point (usually by the fourth hour of the diet), cheats by going on an extraordinary binge,* frequently eating doughnuts at the speed of sound, which is unhealthy.

> *"Guilt is nothing more than repressed anger over the small portions served in expensive restaurants."*

> *"... then, finally, in desperation, I had my jaws wired shut, but they kept popping open."*

---

*Extraordinary binge: Diving face first into Italy.

WHEN DO YOU GO OFF THE BRONX DIET?

To be sure, there will be times when Bronx Dieting is inconvenient or even impossible, but a lapse will not in any way damage your metabolism. Typical non-Bronx Dieting situations include:

- Prison.
- Peace fasts and hunger strikes.
- While skin diving.
- During open heart surgery.
- Vacationing in Borneo.
- Any food-restricted diet.
- Crossing large deserts.
- Coronations.

"Food can be a major weapon in the fight against starvation."

NEW HOPE FOR POOR EATERS

Herbie T., a lumberjack with a nine-inch waist, came to me in desperation. "What can I do?" he asked, "I'm just not that wild about food." Herb explained that he never had a pang when passing a pizzeria, always drained the cheese from his omelets and noshed by sucking oats. To make matters worse, if he didn't finish everything on his plate, his mother spanked his mouth.

"Sit down and have some peanut brittle," I said, and then proceeded to administer the Bronx Diet, a little at a time. First I gently raised his food intake, giving Herb the opportunity to sample the basics—pizza, ice cream and hamburgers. Between meals, because he was not yet ready to snack, I had him "practice" by nibbling brownies.

Three weeks later, Herb's mother wept tears of gratitude when she heard her son ask, for the first time, "Mom, when do we eat?"

"Good peanut butter is like heart cream."

"Better a mangy cupcake than a perfect beet."

NOTICE HOW HAPPILY YOUR BODY RESPONDS

Because the Bronx Diet provides the body with twice the minimal daily adult requirement of everything, there is never a fuel deficiency. Glandular disorders, tongue malformations, and lack of zest become things of the past. Among the physical benefits reported by Bronx Dieters, the most noticeable include:

- Snappier metabolism.
- Lovely bursts of energy.
- Increased verbal skills (especially with the hands).
- Shinier hair and teeth.
- Firmer nails and digits.
- A flatter stomach.
- A more accessible lap.
- Smaller hernias.

"Stillman was the worst. I had to run to the bathroom twice during the third act of Hamlet."
                                              PROMINENT SHAKESPEAREAN ACTOR

THE BITE REPORT: BRONX DIETING AND THE PERFECT RELATIONSHIP

"How do I love thee? Let me count the weighs."

Most Bronx Dieters, in their search for an ideal mate—whether for an evening, a lifetime, or just a little ride on the Ferris wheel—seek not so much a partner as a co-dieter, an eating companion with whom to enjoy civilized weight control. It is for this reason that the Bronx Dieter must choose carefully, lest he or she end up with a vegetarian or, worse, a passive eater who picks at chili and gnaws spare ribs delicately.

Reckless Bronx Dieters have tried relationships based not on eating, but on other common interests such as music, art, and even sex. In most cases, though, these involvements were disastrous, with endless wrangling over tiny portions, risky chicken salad and rigid attitudes toward meat pies.

The importance of holding common eating views was recently emphasized when several hundred Bronx Dieters, as part of a study funded by the National Organization of Eaters (NOE), were asked the question: "Have you ever had food with the opposite sex?" Presented here is a representative sampling of the typical responses.

"Even though she was rich, I married her. She baked perfect garlic bread."

                                        BRONX DIETER WHO FOUND LOVE

"What can you say about a forty-two-year-old bachelor who does Brussels sprouts in a Shake 'n Bake bag?"

                                        PIQUED BRONX DIETER

"For my birthday he gave me a gold locket with a tiny pancake inside."

                                        BRONX DIETER WHO FOUND
                                        A KINDRED SPIRIT

"My husband is so considerate. During sex he bastes my face with ginger ale to keep it from burning."

BRONX DIETER CERTAIN THAT
SHE'S LOVED

"It was terrifying. For a midnight snack she offered two slices of dry Melba toast, eight ounces of skim milk and mashed cauliflower. I pleaded headache, got dressed, and barely made it to the emergency ward of an all-night deli."

BRONX DIETER WHO FOUND HUNGER

"What a head trip! He was way past his eating prime and just getting over two months of Paraguayan cooking, but he still remembered how to make a dish that prolonged you-know-what."

YOUNG BRONX DIETER DATING
AN OLDER MAN

"She calls me her little nosh. In supremely affectionate moments she places tiny wieners in my ears and nibbles them out."

BRONX DIETER WHO FOUND ROMANCE

"We dated for three months and never exchanged a word, possibly because she spoke only Latvian. But it didn't matter since we were mutually fluent in Greek, Spanish, Italian, French, and Finnish food."

HAPPY BRONX DIETER

"How could I not love her? She makes the most deafening stew I've ever tasted, her peach pie is superb, and she's figured out how to turn a Bach cantata into a chocolate cake."

CONTENTED BRONX DIETER

SEX AND THE BRONX DIET

"The morning after that incredible night, we had breakfast in bed. Max served steak, French fries, champagne, and jelly doughnuts. I couldn't tell where the sex left off and the food began."

THROBBING BRONX DIETER

Excellent sex and a buoyant mental outlook permit the Bronx Dieter to indulge in the most taxing, even perverted sexual excesses without so much as a whimper. It is not unusual, in fact, for a Bronx Dieter to enjoy hours of high-octane, nonstop sex without even putting a dent in the heart.

Ordinary diets, however, not only hinder a normal, healthy sex life (the prescribed diet foods often cause the sex organs to oxidize), but actually discourage it. The dieter, having squandered energy on willpower and grating carrots, has just enough strength to sit around waiting for supper. In those rare instances when sex occurs, the debilitated dieter performs at minimal capacity and must constantly be revived with slaps and pinches. Additional sexual problems peculiar to those on regular diets (especially macro- or microbiotic) include:

• Undressing: Dieter too feeble to remove anklets. Must beg understanding partner for assistance.

• Foreplay: Dieter grows aroused only when partner makes carving motions.

• Intercourse: Dieter sustains modest level of excitement by keeping eyes shut and imagining that partner is a *chef de cuisine*.

• Orgasm: Dieter's knee cartilage seldom elastic enough (too many all-beef hot dogs) to allow the necessary movements for a rich, vibrant climax. At best, dieter experiences a "diet" orgasm, which is too low in calories to do any good.

• Post-coital snack: Unleavened herring plus a dish of water.

TRAINING FOR THE BRONX DIET

With most diets, there is a long period of what is known as "deprival training," during which time the dieter, who must go "cold turkey," is instantly cut off from pies, scones, and jug wines. The shock to the system is often so great that many dieters become spur-of-the-moment invalids, able to do little more than salute and use a bedpan.

The Bronx Diet, on the other hand, takes a far less barbaric approach. Referred to by clinicians as "indulgence training," it is a system that by stressing long, slow eating, gradually restores a body ravaged by capricious dieting and builds up tolerance to nourishing, powerful foods.

A more graphic contrast between the two training regimens may be seen on the next page.

"Eating a midnight snack is merely getting the jump on breakfast."

BRONX DIET INDULGENCE TRAINING

(Sample food intake one day before beginning Bronx Diet)

- English muffin with jam
- Omelet
- Doughnut
- Sandwich
- Roast beef hash with corn fritters
- Cheesecake
- Twinkies (one package)
- Potato chips

(Sample food intake first day of Bronx Diet)

- English muffin with less jam*
- Omelet
- Doughnut
- Sandwich
- Roast beef hash *without** corn fritters
- Cheesecake
- Twinkies (one package)
- Potato chip*

*Note implementation of the "to lose, eat less," principle.

ORDINARY DIET DEPRIVAL TRAINING

(Sample food intake one day before beginning ordinary diet)

- English muffin with jam
- Omelet
- Doughnut
- Sandwich
- Roast beef hash with corn fritters
- Cheesecake
- Twinkies (one package)
- Potato chips

(Sample food intake first day of ordinary diet)‡

- One half grapefruit
- Cottage cheese
- Tuna fish
- Tea

‡Note "cold turkey" principle.

DEFYING THE BRONX DIET

Certainly there will be occasions when even the most devoted Bronx Dieter will have curious cravings, not for something sweet or substantial, but rather for grapefruit juice, boiled chicken, and a berry.

No problem.

Statistics show the brownie to be the most popular instrument of diet-breaking. The most popular excuses? "I couldn't help it," "I couldn't hear my heart," and "Nolo contendere" (old Roman excuse).

HOW TO FOLLOW THE BRONX DIET

To feel good, follow the Bronx Diet. To feel better, follow the Bronx Diet Meal Plans.

The Bronx Diet permits weight control without resorting to fads, pills, starvation, or spiritualism. It is the first eating program to take advantage of zero-based dieting, in which medieval diet rules are discarded and the dieter takes personal responsibility for weight control through "Creative Dieting"®—the dieter decides, according to the principles of the Bronx Diet, which foods work best, thus eliminating the middleman. The four essential parts of the Bronx Diet are as follows:

1. EAT WHAT YOU WANT, WHEN YOU WANT IT. This can mean pizza for breakfast, eggs Benedict for lunch, and sirloin steak washed down with a malted for supper. TO REDUCE, EAT LESS: TO GAIN, EAT MORE:* TO MAINTAIN, DO WHATEVER YOU WERE DOING. To those accustomed to the perplexities of counting grams, measuring out ounces, and binging on morsels, these precepts may seem absurdly simple. Yet, millions of happy eaters, including the happy author, are living by these rules and discovering that life can be lemon meringue pies, mounds of lasagna, and handfuls of Hershey Kisses without worrying about weight.

2. USE THE BRONX DIET MEAL PLANS.

"The night I broke up with Marvin, I ate an entire pepperoni pizza, washed it down with some excellent chianti, then tamped the whole thing securely down with a pint of ice cream. Believe me, it was cheaper and far more effective than a month of psychotherapy, and also far less fattening."

LAURA M.

---

*"Eating less" means cutting down on food intake—"Eating more" means increasing food intake.

"Like a fool, I celebrated my wedding 'dietetically'—seven-tiered salad and glasses of tea. Everybody took back their presents. Thank heavens for the Bronx Diet! I just remarried and I assure you that shepherd's pie, champagne, and cream puffs are more fulfilling, more festive and don't alienate guests.

PENELOPE J., REBORN
BRONX DIETER

"I was so depressed when I first moved here. Didn't know a soul and it's so hard to make friends in a big city. The Bronx Diet 'depression' meal plan really helped me. I never before realized how calming a banana split could be."

EZIO P.

"I never thought much of spinach salad for watching a football game."

IGGY J.

The Bronx Diet Meal Plans were developed for the eater who wants to practice weight control while enjoying the healthful benefits of emotional eating. The Meal Plans (pages 106-135), which are based on the correlation between eating and emotional well-being, show the dieter how to use food for everything from enhancing sexual pleasure to exorcising guilt.

While watching a movie, for instance, many Bronx Dieters increase their enjoyment with popcorn and trips to the soda machine; almost all Bronx Dieters agree that an exquisite ending to perfect sex is wine and spaghetti Caruso; and even non-Bronx Dieters know that hot hors d'oeuvres make party guests happier and more inclined to behave.

On a more serious level, Bronx Dieters experiencing emotional distress—anger, guilt, loneliness, boredom, sinus trouble—report even more significant benefits: ten miniature quiches and several chocolate chip cookies eased depression faster than a tin of sauerkraut, pecan pie defused anger quicker than smelts, and one Bronx Dieter actually used meat loaf to successfully make contact with her inner self.

The Bronx Diet gives you sixteen essential Meal Plans, all eater-tested, covering almost any lifelike situation, from infrequent physical contact and feeling sorry for yourself to depression over scrawny plants.

3. INTAKE COMPENSATION. A diet becomes more effective when supplemented by regular physical activity. (It takes eight hours to skip off three pounds of fat.) The Bronx Diet Meal Plans include a series of Intake Compensation Exercise Charts, each prepared according to a corresponding meal plan. Their purpose:

• Guilt-free cheating. Even the most diligent dieter is occasionally seduced by the sight of a handsome popsicle or the aromas emanating from an oven stuffed with ziti. A meal plan calling for one slice of cheesecake may be violated by an enthusiastic dieter who mistakenly eats seven. In either case, there is no need to feel naughty. Simply consult the facing page and select one or all of the exercises to compensate.

• Faster weight loss. If you're not losing fast enough on a particular meal plan, use the exercises to accelerate weight loss. Remember that the more vigorous the exercise, the quicker the weight loss. Hand washing a large building burns off weight much faster than doing a crossword puzzle.

• Slower weight gain. If you went on the Bronx Diet to gain a few pounds and you find you're gaining too fast, simply use the exercises to retard weight gain.

• A firmer, tighter body, more confidence in your grip. Each exercise in Intake Compensation not only promotes weight control, but also improves—more or less—a specific part of your body. For example, if you wish to compensate for a six-inch block of fruitcake and also firm your thighs, you'd refer to the chart and spend one hour roller-skating on a beach. After over-indulging in almond cookies, and for more flexible mouth muscles, a dieter would repeat the phrase *"hochfeines glattes flugpostpapier"* fifty times rapidly. (Cease if you begin to choke.)

4. MUSIC TO EAT BY. The Bronx Diet considers music vital to healthy eating and dieting:

• Digestion. The tranquil effect of Haydn and Mozart upon the pancreas is well-documented. And in many cases, only Beethoven will expedite the internal passage of too much summer sausage.

• Speedier eating. If you're late for work or sleep, a minuet or sprightly gigue will assist the mouth in gobbling down a Danish.

• Music adds to the salubrious effect of food on one's emotional state. A study showed the "Blue Danube" waltz dramatically increased the remedial effect of ice cream in treating parental guilt. One nervous Bronx Dieter discovered that Gregorian chants nearly doubled the calming power of pizza.

• Proper music can make portions seem larger and more robust. Wagner's *Das Rheingold* (uncut) transformed a tuna fish sandwich into a leg of mutton with potatoes and bread pudding.

You will find on each Intake Compensation page a list of musical compositions selected to go with the corresponding meal plan. If you decide to make your own selections, we suggest staying with the classics. Disco precipitates violent intestinal palpitations and polkas cause gas.

TYPICAL BRONX DIET SUCCESS CASE

Webster B.—Male Caucasian, 5′ 10″ 14-month record

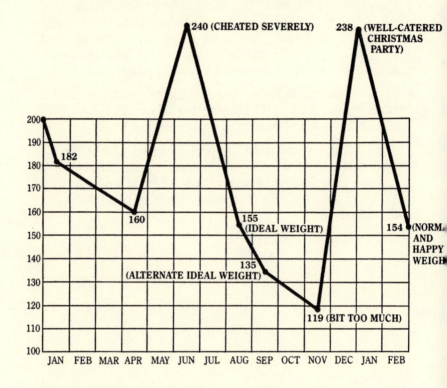

240 (CHEATED SEVERELY)

238 (WELL-CATERED CHRISTMAS PARTY)

182

160

155 (IDEAL WEIGHT)

154 (NORM. AND HAPPY WEIGH

135 (ALTERNATE IDEAL WEIGHT)

119 (BIT TOO MUCH)

JAN FEB MAR APR MAY JUN JUL AUG SEP OCT NOV DEC JAN FEB

MORE SUCCESS STORIES

P.L.—Woman, 5′4″. Followed Dr. Atkins' Diet Revolution for nearly two months but quit when her Ketostix began to explode. Initially skeptical about the Bronx Diet but gave it a chance. Tried the "to reduce, eat less" principle by drastically lowering her yam intake and completely cutting out her usual pre-breakfast snack of oatmeal on a muffin. In just five weeks, she lost 16 pounds and didn't miss them.

BIG JULIUS—Man, 6′1″. Always had huge appetite. Often ate entire chocolate cake in one sitting (or two standings if someone was using the chair). After suffering through 11 diets, he was understandably angry and had bitten his scale into junk. Upon analyzing his eating habits, I discovered that he could easily do without an entire olive loaf each night before retiring. Three weeks later, Medium Julius, 46 pounds lighter, said he felt like "a new man."

J.U.—Man 5'8". Went from 215 pounds to 156 pounds on the Bronx Diet. "My life is now really something. Had to take out a second mortgage to pay the tailoring bills, but it was worth it. I've never been so happy."

H.R.—?, 4'10". "At sixty-three pounds I was laughable. No bust, no waist, no hips, no thighs, no calves, no nothing except very prominent toes. Thank the Lord for the Bronx Diet. I never realized it was so easy to gain weight just by 'eating more.' Now, strangers no longer come up and start petting me."

ONE FAILURE STORY

M.T.—Woman, 5'6". A professional ballet dancer, M.T. was desperate to lose the six pounds gained at her cousin Lenny's wedding. "After two weeks on Stillman, I discovered that due to severe water retention [she had drunk 112 glasses of water but had urinated only twice] I could no longer pirouette; the weight of the water preventing me from getting up on toe." I eliminated her "water block" with beer and then placed her on a strict Bronx Diet regimen, including the meal plan for better sex, just in case. Unfortunately, the poor woman, usually an oral celibate had never sampled so many typical Bronx Diet foods—lasagna, pizza, cheeseburgers with home fried potatoes, Roquefort on pumpernickel, ice cream, potato pancakes, Mounds bars and baked noodles—and completely lost control of herself. Within 5 weeks she had gained 30 pounds, her leotard had burst and her pulse had come to a grinding halt. "I'm still trying," she says.

> *"Fortunately, the recovery rate for most diets is one hundred percent."*

BEFORE BEGINNING THE BRONX DIET

A few pertinent questions:

1. What's wrong with things the way they are now?

2. Do you really want to spend money on a medical checkup? It's how *you* feel that really counts. Many people actually feel worse after a medical checkup, especially if the doctor found nothing wrong.

3. Do you really need a doctor's supervision? In many cases, a caring paramedic, conscientious nurse, or doting mother will do just fine.

4. Are you prepared, for the first time in your life, to go on a diet that gives *you* the responsibility for controlling your weight, or are you a sissy?

5. Are you certain that you're not already on the Bronx Diet?

"I've been on twenty-three diets. All of them worked."
CONFIRMED WAIST-WATCHER

"The way to a man's stomach is through his heart."
DISORIENTED SURGEON

WHAT YOU WILL NEED TO GO ON THE BRONX DIET

LEVEL I PARTICIPATION

1 saucepan
1 large spoon
1 bottle of vitamins
1 hot plate

LEVEL II PARTICIPATION

In addition to several ramekins, you will need:

KNIVES

Large carving knife
Large French chef's knife with
    triangular blade
Slicer
1 or 2 smaller knives for general use
Paring knife
Kitchen scissors
Grapefruit knife

SPOONS

Wooden spoons, various
    sizes
Slotted or perforated spoon
Long-handled spoon for
    basting and stirring large
    amounts of food, such as
    soups
2 or 3 regular kitchen spoons
Measuring spoons
Ladle

FORKS

1 large two-pronged fork
2 or 3 regular kitchen forks
Very small fork for removing
    olives, pickles, etc. from
    small-necked bottles

OTHER TOOLS

Tongs
Wire whisk
Eggbeater
Foodmill or grinder
Pepper grinder
Grater
Potato masher
Lemon squeezer or juicer
Sifter
Sieve
Strainer (colander)
Spatulas (various sizes)
Rubber scrapers
Corkscrew
Can opener
Bottle opener
Apple corer
Vegetable peeler
Vegetable brush
Pastry brush
Rolling pin
Biscuit cutter
Breadboard or work board
Cake rack

DISHES, BOWLS, ETC.

Nest of mixing bowls of various sizes
Wooden chopping bowl with chopper
Measuring cups
Pitcher
1 or 2 kitchen platters
Ovenproof and flameproof serving dishes
Extra dishes and bowls of various sizes

POTS AND PANS

Several saucepans of various sizes
Double boiler
Enamel or glass pan for boiling eggs—they tend to discolor metal pans
Large, deep kettle with tight lid
Dutch oven
Tea kettle
Coffeepot
Medium-sized skillet with lid—heavy cast aluminum, iron, or cast steel are best
Large, heavy skillet with lid
Frying basket for deep-fat frying
Griddle
Several shallow baking dishes, square or oblong, of various sizes

Two or three casseroles of various sizes
Large roasting pan with cover
Loaf pans
Baking sheet
Cake tins
Muffin tins
Pie tins

ALSO

Meat thermometer
Cooking thermometer for deep fat frying

NICE TO HAVE IN· ADDITION

Electric mixing bowl with attachments
Electric blender or puree machine
Electric skillet
Electric deep fryer
Rotisserie
Waffle iron
Steamer with rack
Chafing dish
Omelet pan
Soufflé dishes
Individual pudding cups
Molds
Tube pan for angel food cake and other special cakes
Pastry tube and attachments
Carving board
Poultry shears
Metal skewers

LEVEL III PARTICIPATION

Chef's hat
Electric food processor
Hand-operated ladle

PROPER ATTIRE FOR THE BRONX DIET

One of the problems with most diet plans is the lack of even minimal clothing guidance. Atkins only infers that clothing is low in carbohydrates, Scarsdale counsels white for tennis, and the Canadian Air Force Diet cautions against deep knee bends in leggings.

In the Bronx Diet, we'd like to point out how clothing can help you during mealtimes.

Ideally, of course, meals should be taken in a bathing suit, since human skin is more elastic and stain repellent than gabardine. Since this is seldom possible, we advise, when selecting eating attire, placing the emphasis less on fashion and more on comfort and practicality. Tight French jeans are fine, but after three hours of eating, there will be no pulse below the waist. The following wardrobe tips, if disregarded, will not interfere with weight control.

• Linguine in red clam sauce ruins most ties over four inches long. Instead, wear a bow tie and oilcloth dickey.

• Similarly, it is not a good idea to eat lo-cal borscht in a white silk kimono, especially on a moving bus.

• For picnics, wearing a hat with a long visor (two feet) will protect ice cream from sunburn.

• Always wear a poncho at wine-throwing contests.

• Always wear an amulet to ward off calories.

• Dark soups go better with bold patterns.

• Try to keep your eating pants up to date.

• To ease that "stuffed" feeling, take your shoes off.

• For heavy-duty eating, Scotchgard® your lips.

FOODS PROHIBITED WHEN ON THE BRONX DIET

GROUP I

Okra
Dandelion greens
Broccoli (unless covered by a
    rich sauce)
Turnip greens
Baby food
Di-Gel
Chinese fish
Skim milk

False butter
Boiled eggs
Tripe
Raw bacon
Fatty gelatins
Sandwiches that can be seen
    through when held near a
    candle

GROUP II

Hot dogs containing more
    than 90% cereal filler
Tuna shards
Anything in aspic
Methyl cellulose
Any pill in a candy suspension
Goat's milk
Kosher clams
Boiled duck

Scrapple (unless thoroughly
    washed)
Oats
Bran flakes
Scrod
Ginseng
Wheat germ*
Nacho substitutes

GROUP III

Sake
Canned potato chips
Alfalfa (especially in a sprout
    state)
Well-marbled luncheon meat
Suet
Before-dinner mints
Chewable dessert wines
Chicken beaks

Puddings with a cobalt base
Mood-altering liverwurst
Raw molecules of cake
Frozen knishes covered with
    non-dairy creamer
    (religious ceremony
    excepted)
Any prepackaged bread
    unless an emergency

*Has been found to cause pneumonia in herring.

SKIPPING, A RADICAL CONCEPT

In contrast to most diets, the Bronx Diet allows you to skip any food you don't find agreeable with no adverse side effects!

During a bout with malaria, for instance, a dieter may not be inclined to deal with goat cheese, another dieter may be violently allergic to ham bologna, and several Bronx Dieters insist on the sheer impossibility of synthetic figs.

In addition, the built-in nutritive efficiency of the Bronx Diet permits you to skip *entire meals*,* up to forty in a row, should you lose your job or get lost in the woods.

> *"For the dieter who cheats, the ultimate indignity is having to stop off at a tavern to avoid coming home with telltale chocolate breath."*

---

*Conservative Bronx Dieters, instead of total skipping, may prefer to just pick a little.

SUBSTITUTING

For those who prefer to substitute rather than skip, there's no problem, provided that the dieter exercises common sense.

Food	Acceptable Substitute	Unacceptable
Montrachet in cinders	Brie	Velveeta
Loin of pork	Lamb chops	Spam
Swiss peasant bread	Challa	Zweiback
Fried chicken	Fried shrimp	Gingerbread
Cheesecake	Pecan pie	Taffy
Gnocchi	Potato pancakes	Brussels sprouts
Pâté	Eggplant dip	Minced headcheese
Decadent chocolate cake	Chocolate cake	Decadent parsley
Pizza	—none—	Red English muffins
Antipasto	Ratatouille	Fluffed beet greens

"Avoid foods that rust."

HOW MUCH FOOD SHOULD YOU CONSUME?

Unless you're a contestant, or ravenous, wanton eating is never a good idea—it may lead to hearing voices in the stomach. Many Bronx Dieters learn to "weigh" their food with the eye, or both eyes if they're really hungry, adhering to the motto, "If it looks like enough, it will be enough."

Other Bronx Dieters, however, achieve greater success by practicing portion control with calipers.

The soundest advice, however, is also the simplest: Stop when you've eaten enough to last until the next time.

"Always try to leave something on the table, especially if others are still eating."

WHAT TO DO AS YOU APPROACH YOUR IDEAL WEIGHT

Don't worry.

V. THE BRONX DIET MEAL PLANS

The following sixteen Meal Plans combine the latest in dietetic thinking with discretionary self-indulgence—a system of eating allowing you to enjoy food in the most meaningful ways possible and not just because you're hungry. If you can't find a Meal Plan to match your particular mood or situation, use the Bronx Diet information reaped thus far to create your own.

Note that each sample meal contains a sensible balance of protein, fat, and carbohydrate—all essential building blocks for a total body. But, as mentioned in the "Skipping" and "Substitute" sections, never hesitate to alter a Meal Plan so it fits in better with your new, Bronx Diet way of life.

If, for instance, you feel that green vegetables and fruits have been slighted, don't hesitate to include them. A pea here, a plum there, can't possibly hurt.

Traditionally, most people divide the day's eating into breakfast, lunch, and dinner. In many instances, we have followed this curious system. This does not mean, however, that you must. Any meal can be eaten at any time of the day or, if you prefer, combine breakfast, lunch and dinner into one formidable snack to be eaten, say, between 2:00 and 5:00 A.M.

"Food is the lubricant of the mind."

104 THE BRONX DIET

INDEX TO BRONX DIET MEAL PLANS

Affection 132

Anger 134

Boredom 128

Courage 126

Depression 110

Despair 130

Fatigue 120

Guilt 114

Hangover 124

Healthy Body Heat 136

Insomnia 118

Loneliness 122

Reward 108

Self-Punishment 106

Sex 112

Watching Television 116

"For most dieters, a flannel menu makes the perfect security blanket."

FOOD THERAPY (side view)
How Eating Affects Our Emotional Well-Being
Or Why Eating Makes It All Better

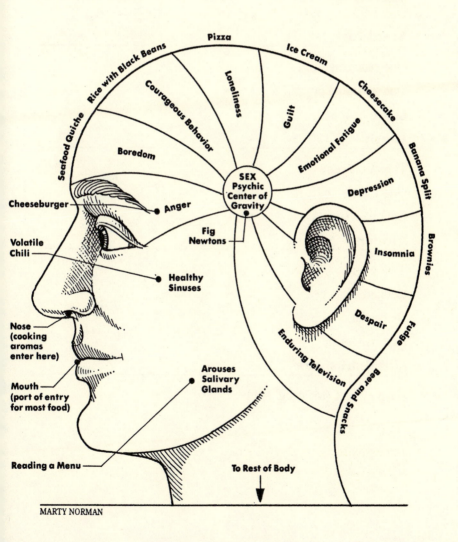

MARTY NORMAN

SELF-PUNISHMENT

Aside from the cathartic effect, a periodic chastening of the
psyche drains off surplus feelings of joy and keeps a well-balanced
life from getting out of hand. Fortunately, for the average, well-
adjusted person, the miracle of modern science has made pain,
suffering, and mortification as close as the nearest non-Bronx
Diet book.

Breakfast

One-half grapefruit

One slice dry protein toast

Coffee or tea

Lunch

Tomato slices

One radish

Coffee or tea

Dinner

Two eggs

Cooked cabbage

Diet gelatin

Diet seltzer

Midnight snack

Dash of suet (for roughage)

INTAKE COMPENSATION

In addition to the meal plan, everyday opportunities to combine weight loss with self-abuse abound, providing the Bronx Dieter with a full range of punishments, from the nearly harmless (chewing Russian-made bubble gum, 60 calories per chew) to the ultimate (spending three months blowing your brains out with a fan burns 145,920 calories). Additional activities:

CALORIES BURNED

Send back your tax return 284

Shave without looking 98

Visit a museum on a crowded Sunday 165

Explore your inner presence by taking your
    chest apart 512

Read an annual report 734

See a veterinarian for your annual checkup 1530

Serve warm beer to a longshoreman 358

MUSIC

Because of the nature of this category, we must take exception to the classical-music-only rule. Instead, we suggest disco with the bass turned up, Albanian rock 'n roll, and atonal hunting cantatas.

REWARD

Why, after performing services above and beyond the call of duty, should you reward yourself with useless trifles? Visiting a dotty uncle, surviving a crash diet, or cleaning out the garage rates more than a pair of new boots and a gold star. Besides, they're inedible. Instead, enjoy a day of sensible, sensuous eating. It's the perfect way to let yourself know that you care.

Breakfast

French toast with raspberry jam

Herb sausages

Chocolate mousse

Coffee, tea, or diet rosé

Lunch

Cold meat loaf

Fried onion rings

Oatmeal cookies

Chilled chablis

Afternoon Cocktail

Cheesecake

Dinner

Caviar

Curried pork

Rice with mushrooms

Edam cheese

Chocolate layer cake

Champagne

Low tar cigar

INTAKE COMPENSATION

Spoil yourself! Take a few days off and fully indulge in your favorite activities. Adventure? Maybe it's finally the time to buy that unicycle and head for parts unknown (264 calories for each part unknown). Self-improvement? How about a perfect tan? (A typical sun worshiper loses three pounds just searching for the ideal tanning position.) Or you can try:

CALORIES BURNED

Tennis: Celebrate your win by jumping
  under the net 174

Golf: Push the golf cart 459
  Carry the caddy 325
  Hit the ball only with the handle of the club 247
  Tee off, then run and see if you can get there
  ahead of the ball..............................798

Jogging: Run a marathon in galoshes..............174

Bowling: Set your own pins 136

Jousting: Use a lead lance and a mule 849

MUSIC

Since all classical music is rewarding, we offer an eclectic choice:

Bizet: *L'Arlésienne:* Suites 1 & 2

Chopin: Études

Purcell: "Ode on St. Cecilia's Day"

Scarlatti: Concerto Grosso no. 4 in E minor

Schumann: String quartet no. 2 in F major (third and fourth movements are perfect while drinking champagne)

DEPRESSION

One of the bouncier meal plans, devised by a psychiatrist and amateur chef who felt the couch took too long. The especial foods contained in this meal plan has made it a favored antidote for dejection, gloom, and profound snits, especially for those not responding to lithium, shock treatment, or a shopping spree.

Wake-up Morsel

Alert the senses with a dish of ice cream. Tamp it down with sponge cake.

Breakfast

Orange juice

Blueberries in whipped cream

Lox, bagels, and cream cheese

Coffee cake

Coffee and chilled Riesling

Lunch

Peanut soup

Cold poached lobster

Large spool of cotton candy
  (optional)

Vanilla malted

Wedge of apple pie

Vodka collins (vital nutritive
  supplement)

Dinner

Miniature quiche

Irish soda bread

Roast duck au Grand Marnier

Baked potato

Marzipan

Chilled chablis or sauterne

Late Night Snack

Chocolate chip cookies

INTAKE COMPENSATION

Combat depression by discovering your own individual strengths. Begin by breaking all of your New Year's resolutions, including the one to go on an all-vinegar diet. Then try:

CALORIES BURNED

Cartwheels in a phone booth (per revolution) 648

10 laps across the bathtub 17

Harpooning the soap 24

Turning over a new leaf:
Maple 2
Oak 3

Leaving your car at home and tricycling to work 269

Clearing your head by jumping on a trampoline
in a room with a six-foot ceiling 85

Also learn inner discipline through yoga: sit cross-legged and knit a sail for your favorite ship

MUSIC

Selected to lift your spirits while you swallow solids.

Beethoven: Ninth Symphony

Berlioz: *Nuits d'été*

Mozart: Concerto in A for Clarinet

Telemann: Concerto in D for 3 Trumpets and 2 Oboes

Vivaldi: Concerto for 4 Violins and Strings in B minor

SEX

"The average orgasm uses seven to eight horsepower per second."

Besides providing the vital nutrients that make things go, food can transform an ordinary sexual experience into something extraordinary—so memorable, in fact, that you may want to frame it. This meal plan supplies the minimum daily adult requirement for long-distance sex (8:00 A.M. to the close of the business day). Those with less time need choose only the meal most appropriate to the particular time of day.

Remember to eat! A day of even moderate sexual activity can burn up to 15,000 calories, which is equivalent to 16 roast chickens or 20 pints of ice cream.

Breakfast

Scrambled eggs with sausages and home fries

Buttered croissants

Gouda cheese

Coffee, tea, or a cordial

Lunch

Yankee bean soup (optional)   Pecan pie

Fried chicken   Chilled chablis or Canadian ale

Ratatouille Niçoise

Afternoon Reviver

Quiche and cream puffs

Dinner

Antipasto   Chocolate-covered cherries

Spaghetti Caruso   Red wine

Lemon meringue pie

INTAKE COMPENSATION

Intensive resting (you've had a hard day)

MUSIC

A control group of Bronx Dieters asserts that the ideal music for sex is chamber music—it provides a rhythm without being intrusive. String quartets by Haydn and Mozart, Schubert's Trio no. 2 in E-flat Major and Beethoven's Quartet no. 5 in A, have helped Bronx Dieters achieve astounding results. For those of you preferring music with more vitamins and minerals:

Mozart: symphonies 36, 40, 41

Delibes: *Coppélia* Suite

Chabrier: *España*

Elgar: "Pomp and Circumstance" (for large partners)

Handel: the *Messiah*

GUILT

Cannoli therapy—the use of food to purge unwarranted guilt—was discovered by a pioneer Bronx Dieter who refused to hate herself after waking at 10:00 A.M. in a married dentist's apartment. Other Bronx Dieters, encouraged by her success, embraced a similar form of treatment, cleansing their souls with everything from Spanish rice with sausages to shepherd's pie and Yoo-Hoo. The following meal plan exculpates all feelings of guilt, unless they come from never calling your parents—then try pâté de campagne and a beaker of slivovitz.

Breakfast

Eggs Benedict

Onion roll with cream cheese and jelly

Pecan ring

Coffee, tea, or a Pepsi

Lunch

Hot roast beef sandwich

Macaroni salad (or sandwich)

Blueberry pie with French vanilla ice cream

Half bottle of Bordeaux (red or white, decent year)

Dinner

Saddle of lamb

Roast potatoes, plenty of gravy

Corn bread

Peach pie

Champagne or V-8 juice

INTAKE COMPENSATION

For best results, weight loss activities should be whole-somely sinful, allowing you to flaunt your new psychic strength. Try some good, healthy anonymous sex, perhaps with someone who just dented your car (438 calories). Or, if you don't happen to drive:

CALORIES BURNED

Take apart Daddy's watch	30

Cheerlead:

Pulling on white boots	16
Twirling a baton (per twirl)	2
Learning the cheers	457
Shaking your pompon	77
Turning down a football player	1

Do charity work (for yourself)	100
Violate human rights (per right)	28
Buy a new hat with the rent money	42
Cheat a trusting soul	56

MUSIC

To cleanse the soul, listen to:

Brahms: First Symphony

Mahler: Second Symphony

Grofé: *Grand Canyon* Suite

Holst: *The Planets*

Borodin: "Polovetsian Dances"

WATCHING TELEVISION

In many cases, a selection of carefully chosen food will enhance an already first-rate show. "Tom and Jerry," "Popeye," and the "Uncle Floyd Show," for instance, are even better with a delicate white wine and five authentic nachos. For other, less amusing programs, however, remaining still for 30 or more minutes will demand at least a large sandwich and two bottles of high-cal beer. For a one-hour special featuring a singing family, a six-course snack is indispensable. A poll of Bronx dieting video fans throughout the United States suggests the following foods:

Program Category	Suggested Food Choices
Educational Television	Red wine, Roquefort cheese, yogurt, pâté en croute, smoked salmon, white caviar salad, dried fruits, marzipan, Swedish meatballs
Game Shows	Popcorn, any E-Z spread cheese on Ritz crackers, Pepsi-Cola, crunchy pickles, bubble gum, Skippy peanut butter, potato chips (unridged), Ring Dings, Yankee Doodles, Devil Dogs, leftover tuna fish casserole, can of sardines, sloppy Joes
Soap Operas	Brownies, entire Whitman Sampler, potato salad, chicken salad sandwich, fudge, Mallomars, ice cream, salami, grilled American cheese on toast, Dr. Pepper
Old Movies (especially on Sunday afternoon)	Beer or wine, fried chicken (order out from local chicken emporium), McDonald's, pizza, pecan or cherry pie, Jarlsberg or Gruyère cheese, peanut brittle
Talk Shows	Cold meat loaf, white wine, red wine, chocolate cake, blintzes, provolone cheese, crab cakes, Three Musketeers, German liverwurst on pumpernickel, and beer

Situation Comedies	Hard liquor
Made-for-TV Movies	Muscatel

INTAKE COMPENSATION

Vigorous channel changing

Constantly adjusting the color tone

MUSIC

Superfluous

INSOMNIA

Unless sleeplessness has a tangible cause—seasickness, a crowded bed, a meal that's backfiring—chances are good that eating the proper foods will induce healthy slumber.* Be sure to eat all meals within falling distance of a bed, should the food take effect without warning.

Breakfast

Cheese soufflé

Bialy with marmalade

Hot chocolate with dash of Kahlúa

Lunch

Turkey and pastrami on rye with cole slaw and Russian dressing

Home-prepared potato salad

Two bottles of beer and/or 16-oz. flagon of wine

Dinner

Prosciutto and melon

Big pile of gnocchi

Banana cream pie

Hogshead of sangría (not on a school night)

Midnight Snack (skip if you're asleep)

Fudge

* The heavier the food, the deeper the sleep. An anchovy will, at best, produce a fitful doze. Manicotti, on the other hand, induces a restful coma, complete with snoring.

INTAKE COMPENSATION
Activities should be gentle and as bed-oriented as possible.

CALORIES BURNED

Getting into bed	12
Lying still, awaiting sleep	26
Growing impatient	34
Tossing and turning	47
Fluffing up the pillows	15
Smoothing the blanket	19
Again lying still, awaiting sleep	26
Staring up at the ceiling	10
Staring down at the pillow	14
Both at the same time	1593
Counting sheep (per sheep)	18
(Using a pocket calculator)	11

MUSIC
Noted for tranquillity and serenity are:

Bach: Sonatas and Partitas for Unaccompanied Violin

Mozart: *Eine Kleine Nachtmusik*

Debussy: *La Mer*

Schubert: Quintet in A

Brahms: Trio in E flat for Horn, Violin, Piano

Wagner: Anything. Among composers, Wagner holds the record for putting people to sleep.

FATIGUE

Excessive weariness after a nine-hour tax audit, collapsing from jet lag, and that Monday morning drained feeling after a surprisingly intensive weekend are nothing to worry about, unless they happen all at once. Your body is simply exhausted and needs time to mend. The first step is to conserve strength by not going to work. Call in tired and devote the day to resting, sitting in a chair, reading and talking to friends on the telephone. Next, rebuild the body and elate the mind with prudent eating. Actually preparing and eating "meals" will be tiring and, in your weakened state, you probably won't be able to keep track of which comes first: dinner, midnight snack, breakfast, high tea, or lunch. Instead, keep a selection of the following foods nearby, all of which contain energy and require minimal skills. Eat as needed.

Brazil nuts	Reputable pepperoni pizza
Eggplant dip	Macaroni salad
Stuffed figs	Cheese Doodles
Carrot bread	Necco wafers
Banana bread	Peanut butter and jelly on a bran muffin
Molasses cookies	Ice cream sundae
Riboflavin	Walnut pie
Toffee bars	Gefilte fish
Nestlé's Crunch bars	Cupcakes
Corned beef on rye	Mason Dots

INTAKE COMPENSATION

For obvious reasons, activities should be light, yet dynamic enough to compensate for molasses cookies. Weaving garlands, fine-tuning your radio, coughing, and studying your face all help keep your weight down, and you don't have to reserve a court. Other light, but substantial activities include:

CALORIES BURNED

Flexing your toes 15

Dusting small objects (a child, for instance) 34

Drumming fingers on a hotplate 86

Stringing Cheerios 21

Practicing your signature 3

Light housekeeping 57

Light sex (keep shoes, watch, and sweater on) 125

MUSIC

Avoid music that might tire the ears and weary the brain. We suggest:

Albinoni: Adagio for Strings and Organ

Barber: Adagio for Strings

Beethoven: Adagio and Allegro for Music Box

Mozart: Adagio in C for Glass Harmonica
Adagio for 2 Clarinets and 3 Basset-Horns

Schubert: Adagio and Rondo concertante in F

Schumann: Adagio and Allegro for Horn

LONELINESS

No matter what the reasons—Saturday night and no date ...
a recent transfer to Guam ... quarantined for life ... congeni-
tally obnoxious personality ... banished by the king—you're
never alone with food nearby, since it represents the ultimate in
passive companionship. Many Bronx Dieters, in fact, prefer the
company of above-average food to below-average people. A
roasted squab never tells its life story and you don't have to wait
until the manicotti leaves to go to bed.

Breakfast

3 flapjacks with New England maple syrup

Swiss cheese omelet with bacon

6 Pepperidge Farm Milanos

Coffee, tea, or a milkshake

Lunch

Special "friend" sandwich (a Bronx Diet first): Slice a 30-inch loaf
of French bread lengthwise, dig a trench in both sides, and fill to
brimming with either good pâte or salami, ham, and provolone
cheese. Combine all four if you can take it. Talk nicely to your
sandwich, it will respond.

Afternoon Pick-Me Up

Pizza with extra cheese, meatballs, sausages, mushrooms,
green peppers, and onions

Dr. Brown's Cel-Ray Tonic

Dinner

Homemade French onion or thick and hearty pea soup. (Note:
making soup from a can diminishes its companion value by half.)

Country ham with apricots and pineapple rings

Wild rice (be good to yourself, even if you have to take out a
mortgage to pay for the rice)

Brownie al dente

Medium-price red Bordeaux

Midnight Snack

Napoleon

INTAKE COMPENSATION

To combine a feeling of companionship with weight loss, spend the evening crashing parties. The more exclusive the affair, the more calories burned. Just pushing your way past a hulking Pinkerton guard can remove up to 300 calories, which more than makes up for the wild rice and the brownie al dente. If crashing isn't your style try:

A singles bar: CALORIES BURNED

Getting up the nerve to ask someone if you can
   buy them a drink (the bartender, for instance) 84

Getting up the nerve to ask someone if they'll
   buy you a drink 268

If you don't like singles bars:

Press a glass against the wall and listen to your
   neighbors argue 23

Join the army 136

MUSIC

For an evening of congeniality we suggest two operas: *The Barber of Seville* or *Die Fledermaus*, which is a musical New Year's Eve party. If you're not enchanted with opera, try:

Mozart: Piano concerti nos. 19, 20, 21, 25, 27

Rimsky-Korsakov: *Scheherazade*

Handel: *Water Music*

Saint-Saëns: *Carnival of the Animals*

HANGOVER

Bronx Dieters know that the only remedy for a hangover is sitting still and hoping it will pass. During this time, which may last several weeks, the dieter must take some sort of nourishment. To prevent accidents, however, foods ingested should have a low atomic weight. Ice cream, raisin bread, and apricot nectar are excellent, since they stimulate the pineal gland to fight off nausea should the dieter sneeze. The following list, while by no means definitive, represents foods to avoid until recovery is complete.

Squid

Bread pudding

Rumanian goulash

Chili burritos

Stuffed flank steak

Scallops in horseradish

Oyster stew

Lamb stew

Headcheese

Bavarian-style bloodwurst

Puréed shrimp

Hard-boiled eggs

Knockwurst

Hot dog tips

Moussaka

Lentil soup

Spinach quiche

Warm vodka

ACTIVITIES TO AVOID

Sit-ups

Canoe rides

Breathing bus exhaust

Abrupt turns

Hanging drapes

Changing kitty litter

Pie-eating contests

Figure skating

Baton twirling

Rain dancing

MUSIC TO AVOID

Wagner: "Ride of the Valkyries"

Botticelli: Concerto for Sousaphone, Saxophone, and Strings

Mendoza: Bugle Calls of the Mexican Army

Mussorgsky: "Night on Bald Mountain"

Marches: "Thunder and Blazes," "The Mad Major," "Colonel Bogey," "2nd Regiment Connecticut National Guard," "National Emblem," "Lights Out," and "The Washington Post"

COURAGE

Valorous deeds demand spirited foods—imagine declaring war or returning a bathing suit bolstered by nothing but half a grapefruit and a chicken wing. Bronx Dieters are well acquainted with the fortifying powers of foods. One individual, after consuming $68.47 worth of Hungarian goulash, actually had the nerve to ask for a raise he didn't deserve. Another Bronx Dieter, a former wimp, proposed marriage to a woman of higher station after eating just one bowl of West Indian hot and pungent turkey fricassee, a dish listed as a controlled substance in parts of the Midwest. And before blind dates, one woman—as a matter of course—takes a heaping spoonful of kumquats.

Breakfast

Screwdriver   Black currant jam

Ham and eggs   10 Black Crows

Buttermilk pancakes

Lunch

Sausage and hot peppers on Italian bread

Limburger cheese (dare to have aggressive breath)

Dark beer

Dinner

Yankee bean soup (homemade, of course)

Linguine with red clam sauce

Linguine with white clam sauce

Italian cheesecake

Red burgundy

Intrepid snack

Cuchifritos

INTAKE COMPENSATION

Activities should test one's mettle in preparation for bigger things. Debuting on roller skates in downtown traffic, for instance, burns 567 calories, add 50 more calories if you don't know how to stop. Presenting a summons to a policeman for jaywalking is also good (79 calories). Also try:

CALORIES BURNED

Hang gliding by your thumbs 81

Hang gliding by someone else's thumbs 562

Escaping from prison (medium security) 1479

Picking a stranger's nose........................ 55

Wearing a derby during sex..................... 78

Insulting a Mexican border guard 345

MUSIC

Heroic compositions include:

Bach: Mass in B minor

Beethoven: *Wellington's Victory*

Haydn: Symphony no. 100 (*Military*)

Rossini: *William Tell* Overture

Tchaikovsky: *1812* Overture

Von Suppé: Overtures

BOREDOM

Nothing on television? Barren social life? Amusement park closed? Best friend speaks only Welsh? Getting through the day can be arduous, especially if you rise at 4:00 A.M. Fortunately, with food around, there's never a problem. Among Bronx Dieters, eating to fill time is a common practice—a nourishing way to keep out of mischief, occupy the hands, and stimulate creativity.

Breakfast

Fried rice

Apple muffins

Choice of spare ribs or venison stew

Fresh orange juice with anisette

Lunch

Grilled cheese and bacon on challah

Candied sweet potatoes

Homemade apple strudel (preparation alone takes up to four hours)

Carafe of California chablis

Dinner

Steak tartare

Minestrone

Banana split (five-scooper)

White burgundy

Midnight Snack

Cadbury hazelnut bar

INTAKE COMPENSATION

Unorthodox silliness and total self-amusement is the rule
for these activities.

CALORIES BURNED

Jumping rope while wearing scuba flippers 87

Achieving eye contact with an adult giraffe 123

Eating rice in a wind tunnel 455

Any tug of war with a hostile nation 1596

Boiling large articles of furniture 275

Another way to pass the time and compensate for lunch is
isometric sex, which burns off 516 calories per hour.

MUSIC

Compositions you can really sink your ears into include:

Beethoven: Military band music

Berlioz: *Harold in Italy*

Haydn: Symphony no. 51 (during the second movement, it is
customary to show reverence for the horn player by holding a
fork across one's chest)

Prokofiev: *Peter and the Wolf*

Vivaldi: Concerto in G for 2 Mandolins

DESPAIR

The following meal plan comes from an eminent Bronx Dieter—
the co-inventor of the precrumpled handbill—who one day discovered that his world visibly brightened after two honey crum-
pets and a flagon of cider. Other Bronx Dieters report rapid relief
from melancholy with a variety of foods, ranging from a well-
turned turkey leg to wild kasha. If you've lost all hope of master-
ing that intricate dance step, winning a contest, or becoming the
person your parents meant you to be, try the following meal plan,
several times a day if necessary.

Breakfast

Waffles with ice cream   Coffee, tea, or Royal Crown Cola

Waldorf salad   Hot bath

Lunch

Oysters Rockefeller

Green peas cooked in butter

Potato pancakes with applesauce

Peanut butter fudge

Chilled liebfraumilch

High Tea

Noodle pudding

Dinner

Clams on the half shell

Chicken breasts stuffed with spinach, pâté, and zucchini

Hash brown potatoes

Apple pie with ice cream of choice

Beer or wine (plenty of it)

INTAKE COMPENSATION

Seek cheery ways to pass the time and divert your mind. A brisk walk through a china shop with your arms outstretched (76 calories), sneaking into a movie (90 calories), or making funny faces at passing strangers (24 calories per face) are popular among formerly despondent Bronx Dieters. Also do good deeds:

CALORIES BURNED

Volunteer to open stuck windows for the elderly
  (per stuck window) 45

Sell your house for a nickel 258

Help an old car across the street...................429

Become the town crier (per cry)................. 46

Steal from the rich and keep most of it 173

Deprogram a Moonie 816

MUSIC

Delius: *Florida* Suite (perfect music for chicken breasts)

Sibelius: *Finlandia*

Schumann: Symphony no. 1

Handel: *Alexander's Feast*

Mozart: *The Marriage of Figaro*

AFFECTION

Got a splitting heartache? Lover inert during sex? Feeling rejected by insensitive siblings? Stop sniveling and start eating. Turning to food is a perfectly healthy way to get what you need when it's not available through normal channels. A tender dalliance with a fruit cake or a few Hershey Kisses will more than compensate for a withholding lover or the cold shoulder from your dog.

Breakfast

Maypo

Stack of wheat cakes with plenty of syrup

Apricot or cheese Danish

Chocolate milk

Lunch

Ziti salad   Italian cheesecake

Two slices of Sicilian pizza   Carafe of dry red wine

Low Tea

Hot fudge sundae

Frozen Daiquiri

Dinner

Sliced Westphalian ham on melon

Eggplant parmigiana

Spaghetti in homemade sauce

Strawberry shortcake

Chianti with a side of beer

Midnight Snack

Chocolate rum ball

INTAKE COMPENSATION

	CALORIES BURNED
Hugging a meat loaf	49
Kissing soup	25
Sleeping with a muffin	18
Fondling gnocchi	36
Petting a cheeseburger	19
Caressing beef	60
Whispering endearments into a chicken's ear	15
Cuddling cheese	54
Cherishing a flapjack	21

MUSIC

Five affectionate pieces to satisfy the lovelorn:

Bach: Cantata 147

Beethoven: Sonata no. 5 for Violin & Piano

Mozart: Quartets nos. 20 & 21

Puccini: *La Bohème*

Schubert: *Die schöne Müllerin*

ANGER

Anthropologists tell us that primitive peoples vented anger by chewing rocks. Early Bronx Dieters, when angry, chewed untenderized chuck steak. Today, new advances in eating make such extremes unnecessary. Coping with the major problems of our society—insolent waiters, judgmental hairdressers, long bank lines, and children's portions in adult restaurants—is easy with the following, scientific meal plan.

Breakfast

Apricot dumplings (very good for gnashing teeth)

Sharp cheddar or Stilton cheese

Oatmeal and raisin cookies

Espresso

Lunch

Rock candy

Italian olive salad

Shish kebab (gnaw on the skewer)

Rice pilaf

Dark beer or two martinis

Dinner

Chicken parmigiana

Spaghetti with garlic

Garlic bread

Halvah or pecan pie

Dry vermouth or red wine (try an Algerian red if you feel feisty)

INTAKE COMPENSATION

Exercise anger away with martial sports such as judo, karate, and Christmas shopping. Less taxing but effective are:

CALORIES BURNED

Temper tantrums:
Lying on floor and kicking legs in air 68

Standing up and kicking legs in air
(both at the same time) 303

"Taking it out" on your spouse 72

Terrorizing a parakeet 45

Parallel parking your car at 45 mph 248

Punching a stallion unconscious 419

MUSIC

To soothe the savage breast—and a possible savage stomach:

Chopin: Mazurkas

Mendelssohn: Symphony no. 4 *(Italian)*

Pachelbel: "Kanon"

Rossini: Sonatas for Strings

Tchaikovsky: *Sleeping Beauty*

Vivaldi: *Four Seasons*

HEALTHY BODY HEAT

Although not for psychic relief in the strictest sense, our Bronx
Diet advisory panel felt that uncertain oil supplies, lower ther-
mostat settings, and an impending ice age made this category
essential to dieters residing more than 30 miles from the equator.
Gourmet eaters will, of course, instantly recognize this regimen
as an elaborate version of the Eskimo technique for keeping
warm: a no-frills meal plan consisting of blubber and snow.

Breakfast

Hot oatmeal with raisins

Spiced gefilte fish

Corn muffins with melted butter

Coffee, tea, or mulled wine

Lunch

Lentil soup

Curried lamb with green mango pickle

Rice

Two tots of rum

Dinner

Guacamole dip

Swiss fondue

All-purpose chili (if prepared correctly, should make the back of
your head sweat profusely)

Irish coffee or Irish tea

Midnight Snack

Indoor clambake

INTAKE COMPENSATION

The harder you work, the warmer you become and the more calories burned. Taking the dog for a brisk walk burns 120 calories, more if it doesn't want to go. If you don't have a dog, steal a neighbor's or else attach a leash to a log and drag it down the street. (Burn 40 extra calories by carrying your own fireplug.) If you have a green thumb, planting a garden, especially on a sidewalk, can burn over 800 calories in just a few short minutes. Other lighter, but effective activities include reshingling a birdhouse (27½ calories), installing a basketball net without using a ladder (88 calories), and helping the mailman (73 calories).

MUSIC

Lively gigues and perky symphonies are good for the blood. With the right music, in fact, you won't need woolen underwear.

Chopin: Waltzes

Handel: *Royal Fireworks Music*

Stravinsky: *Firebird* Suite

Offenbach: *Gaîté Parisienne*

Beethoven: Fifth Symphony

Schubert: Minuets

THE BRONX DIETER'S GUIDE TO DINING OUT

"What you eat is more important than who you'll meet."

DINNER PARTIES: It is safe to assume that the portions will be small, especially if your host is wealthy. The Bronx Dieter naive enough to arrive hungry will spend much time in the bathroom, trying to quell hunger pangs with toothpaste. Always take the precaution of eating before going out to dinner.

THE INFORMAL PARTY: Affords the dieter greater eating freedom, especially while the other guests are dancing. This does not mean, however, ignoring the rules of sensible nutrition. A few tips:

1. Keep up your strength by staying close to the food table (lean against it, if you have to). Additional advantages of this strategy include:

- *Meeting most of the guests*

- *Discovering whom to avoid*

- *First chance at new dishes as they're brought to the table*

2. Avoid the inexpensive cheeses: domestic Swiss, Argentine Gouda, Wisconsin "Roquefort," Velveeta, and questionable dips.

3. The same applies to cold cuts. Bologna, olive loaf, luncheon meat, and Spam are eerie meats better fit for a child's lunchbox.

4. Ham, prosciutto, roast beef, and other, more aristocratic meats should be eaten right away, before they are spotted by the other guests. If you're temporarily full, put a selection in your pockets for later.

5. When not eating, dance vigorously. Twenty minutes of bouncing compensates for a turkey on rye with mustard.

6. Eat balanced snacks. Don't be afraid to check your hosts' refrigerator to see if they've held anything back.

7. When taking refreshment, never immerse face totally in the punchbowl. If there's no ladle, cup your hands.

8. It is safer to use your fingers when eating rollable foods such as midget wieners, meat balls and grapes.

9. Don't carp about the food until you're full, and nearly ready to leave.

RESTAURANTS: Explain that you're on the Bronx Diet; they'll usually be happy to accommodate you. Remember, however, that French restaurants conceal small portions under layers of sauce. Italian restaurants employing a tuxedoed maitre d' with wavy hair are risky, and walk quickly past Chinese restaurants with bread on the table. Safest are Chinese restaurants without tablecloths, Italian restaurants with paper place mats featuring the points of interest in Cremona, and any pizzeria with several outstanding health citations.

Also, before entering any restaurant, consider these points:

1. Is there a menu in the window? If not, what are they trying to hide?

2. Jacket and tie required? If so, the management obviously takes more of an interest in fashion than in food. Avoid.

3. Study the waiters. Are they thin? Do they shamble along, muttering to themselves? Do they bring their own lunch?

4. Study the patrons. Are there any?

5. Are the tables huddled together? Nearby eaters may communicate harmful bacteria or, worse yet, may snitch your food.

6. Is there a cover charge for silverware?

WHEN TRAVELING: In foreign countries, follow these simple rules:

• Thoroughly wash all fruit, even if it's already in your pie.

• Be wary of duck in Yemen.

• Never drink wine from the tap.

- Never eat a sandwich that you find on the street.

- Steak tartare in Uganda is risky.

- Avoid exotic concoctions—green tapioca, Siamese meatballs, creamed oats—you may stop resembling your passport photo.

"Within seven days of leaving a reducing spa, ninety percent of all former patients are stopped for speeding while driving to the bakery."

EPILOGUE: FINAL THOUGHTS FOR THE BRONX DIETER

- Never eat with your mouth full.
- Beware of vegetarians.
- Beware of people who eat only when hungry.
- Avoid restaurants with "natural" in their name.
- Ditto "organic" and "health."
- Greasy pork chops are a vital source.
- Chocolate cake will see you through a harrowing toboggan ride better than a sourball.
- Eating is not a science—listen to your mouth.
- Inside every diet doctor is a pastry chef screaming to get out.
- Never order pastrami in a Chinese restaurant.
- There's no shame in fighting for an advantageous position at a formal buffet, even if you're the ambassador.
- Never eat by candlelight—you may stick a fork in your forehead.
- Perfect macaroni salad is a rarity—protect it in a refrigerated safety deposit box.
- Never insert your face in a stranger's picnic basket.
- It's hard to get wasted on pan-broiled liver.

"There's more than one way to skin a grapefruit, but who cares?"

BIBLIOGRAPHY

Dietrich, Clancy. *Tiefgefrorenes Mussen Sie Aber Vor Dem Servieren Auftauen*. Stuttgart: Autobahn Press, 1978.

Dostoevski, Fëdor. *The Brothers Karamazov*. New York: The New American Library, Inc. 1881.

Dutzberg, Thorton. *I'll Diet Tomorrow*. International Archives of Eating, Vol. 56, No. 4, 1974.

Feldman, Leroy. "They Done Nabbed My Kasha." Unpublished Ph.D. Dissertation, Department of Anthropology, Jake's University, 1977.

Gravy, J. T. *Dieting in the Court of Henry VIII*, Vol. 3. London: Stonehenge Press, 1954.

Harvey, Jeff. "Whatever Happened to the Creamsicle?" New Jersey: Personal Letter, 1972.

Histadrut, Gaylord. "Eclair Deprivation in Warriors." *Congressional Record*, Vol. 119, No. 90, 1973.

Sudliff, Henry. *Behavioral Patterns in Chicken Fondling*. Virginia: Ozark Publishing House, 1978.

Teawurst, Herschel. "Junk Food, Junk Sex—Which is Merrier?" New York City: Food Museum Bulletin No. 4, 1976.

Verdi, Giuseppe. *La Traviata*, 1853.

"Buddha wasn't much of a dieter either."